HEALING
DIABETES

HEALING
DIABETES

Complementary Naturopathic
& Allopathic Treatments

DR ALEXANDER McLELLAN, ND
& DR MICHAËL FRIEDMAN, ND
WITH JENNIFER LEMON, RHN

CCNM
PRESS

The authors thank Jennifer Lemon for her practical dietary information and recipes. Thanks also to Judyth Moulson for her work on the Dietary Therapy chapter. Mostly thanks to our patients without whom this book would not have been possible.

The publisher does not advocate the use of any particular treatment program, but believes that the information presented in this book should be available to the public. The nutritional, medical, and health information presented in this book is based on the research, training, and personal experiences of the authors, and is true and complete to the best of their knowledge. However, this book is intended only as an informative guide for those wishing to know more about good health. It is not intended to replace or countermand the advice given by the reader's physician. The publisher and the authors are not responsible for any adverse effects or consequences from any of the suggestions made in this book. Because each person and each situation is unique, the publisher and the authors urge the reader to consult with a qualified professional before using any procedure where there is any question as to its appropriateness.

ISBN 1-897025-16-5

Edited by Bob Hilderley.
Design by Sari Naworynski.

Printed and bound in Canada.

Published by CCNM Press Inc., 1255 Sheppard Avenue East,
Toronto, Ontario M2K 1E2 Canada.
www.ccnmpress.com

BRIEF CONTENTS

DESCRIPTIVE CONTENTS

Quick Reference Guide to Diabetes,

Disorder	Major Signs and Symptoms	Key Tests
Diabetes Type I	Weight loss	High glucose High glycosylated hemoglobin High fructosamine levels
Diabetes Type II	Obesity	High glucose High glycosylated hemoglobin High fructosamine levels
Hypoglycemia	Irritable when missing meals	None
Hyperinsulinemia	Acanthosis nigracans (darkening of the skin) Obesity	High insulin levels Possibly high glucose levels
Syndrome X	High or normal blood glucose, High triglycerides, Low HDL High blood pressure Skin tags Truncal fat deposits	Glucose insulin tolerance test (GITT) - high insulin levels Serum lipids
Diabetic Retinopathy	None or blurred vision or 'floaters'	Visual acuity test Dilated eye exam Tonometry
Diabetic Neuropathy	Numbness, burning, tingling, and pain in the extremities	Pin prick, sensation, vibration sense testing Nerve conduction testing Glycosylated hemoglobin
Diabetic Nephropathy	None in early stages Later fatigue, frothy urine, headache, swelling around the eyes in the mornings	Urine protein Blood pressure Serum creatinine and BUN
Gestational Diabetes	None or increased thirst, increased urination, fatigue, frequent infections, blurred vision	Fasting glucose Glucose tolerance test

Prediabetic Conditions, and Diabetic Complications

Conventional Therapies	Naturopathic Therapies
Insulin	Insulin Diet and nutritional supplements to prevent disease and diabetic complications
Sulfonylureas Biguanides	Botanical medicines, low glycemic diet, nutritional supplements, exercise
None	Botanical medicines, nutritional supplements, adrenal support, stress management
Biguanides	Botanical medicines, low glycemic diet, chromium, vanadium, exercise
Symptom management with diuretics, antihypertensives, and cholesterol lowering drugs	Botanical medicines, low glycemic diet, nutritional supplements, exercise
Pharmaceutical management of blood sugar and lipids Laser surgery for proliferative forms	High dose antioxidants,bioflavanoids (lutein), IV glutathione
Neurontin Lyrica Cymbalta	Topical botanical medicines, low glycemic diet, nutritional supplements, exercise
Antihypertensives	High dose antioxidants,botanical kidney tonics, blood sugar balancing, nutritional supplements
Diet and exercise Insulin injection	Low glycemic diet, chromium supplementation, exercise, small regular meals

Naturopathic Medical Outcomes

Naturopathic medicine has proven to be effective in many cases for preventing and treating Type I and Type II diabetes, prediabetic conditions, and diabetic complications.

Type I Diabetes

Several naturopathic therapies, including intravenous hydrogen peroxide, niacinamide, and neuropeptide injections upon diagnosis, have shown a positive effect in promoting remission, lowering insulin requirements, and increasing beta cell function. There are a few reported cases of completely eliminating exogenous insulin with the use of natural medicine. Naturopathic approaches to diabetic management also play an important role in reducing the risk of diabetic complications.

Following naturopathic protocols:
- Some recently diagnosed Type I patients may go into complete remission.
- Patients can more tightly control blood glucose levels.
- Patients can often decrease insulin requirements and reduce dependence on exogenous insulin.
- Patients can improve quality of life through the prevention of complications that can range from mild to debilitating.

Type II Diabetes

Studies have shown that only about 25% of diabetic patients on oral diabetic medicine are able to achieve good (not perfect) control of their blood sugar levels. However, many patients who are treated with naturopathic medicine are able to maintain good blood sugar control without the need for pharmaceutical medicines for diabetes Type II. As with pharmaceutical hypoglycemic agents, there are always some individuals who do not respond.

Following naturopathic protocols:
- Blood sugar can begin to decrease within 2 weeks, but it may take 6 weeks before some people notice a change. Approximately 88%

of people are able to lower their blood sugar levels within 3 months of continued use, based on clinical research of herbal combinations containing jambul and devil's club.

- Patients with excessive insulin can expect about a 30% decrease in 3 months. After 2 months of daily use, most people will notice a decrease in blood sugar.
- Fasting blood sugar should go down within 8 weeks and HBA1c values within 3 months.

Side Effects

Reported adverse side effects from use of naturopathic diabetic nutrient and botanical medicines are rare.

Drug Interactions

The medicinal nutrients and herbs used in naturopathic approaches to preventing and treating diabetes balance blood sugar, so there is little possibility of blood sugar going too low when conventional drugs are used in combination with naturopathic medicines.

Weaning Off Drugs

Once patients following naturopathic protocols start to notice a significant decrease in blood sugar levels, they can consider starting to wean themselves off any prescription drugs they may be taking for their condition. Some people may be able to start weaning after 2 weeks of following naturopathic protocols, while others may be able to start after 8 weeks. It is not recommended for patients to stop their prescription drugs when their blood sugars are consistently over 150 mg/dL.

Side Benefits

Many naturopathic nutrients and herbs can help eliminate free radicals, which are largely responsible for the secondary complications of diabetes. Secondary complications of diabetes might get better while following naturopathic protocols. Vision and kidney function might improve.

INTRODUCTION

Diabetes is most succinctly explained as a disease that affects the way in which our bodies convert the food we eat into energy. In a healthy individual, this conversion would be made efficiently with the help of insulin, a hormone produced in the pancreas that enables glucose molecules from food to pass through cell membranes so that it can be used as energy or stored for the future. If you or someone you know has diabetes, it means that either there isn't sufficient insulin for this conversion to occur or that, for some reason, the insulin is not eliciting a response in the body. Either way, the result is unstable blood sugar levels, which can soar dangerously high and lead to severe diabetic complications or even death.

Although stress, exercise, and stimulants can all affect blood sugar levels, food is usually the most significant concern for diabetics because it can raise blood sugar sharply and often immediately, and its consumption is a necessary part of daily life. Given that we live in a society where food is not only abundantly available, but also abundant in calories, the significance of a blood sugar disorder cannot be overstated.

Diabetes Epidemic

B efore the discovery of insulin in the early 1920s by Dr Frederick Banting and Dr Charles Best, diabetes was a fatal disease with no known methods of treatment or prevention. Their discovery has since led to a rash of research into the mechanisms of diabetes, its management, and the possibility of a cure. In 2004, more than $36 million was invested in research by the American Diabetes Association alone, almost doubling its financial research support from 5 years prior. These sorts of investments have generated many new possibilities for the prevention and management of diabetes.

However, the prevalence of diabetes continues to rise, burdening our healthcare system with exploding costs. The World Health Organization predicts that diabetes will be one of the worst killers in the world by the year 2025, affecting some 300 million people worldwide. Diabetes is already costing American taxpayers $132 billion every year, representing $1.00 out of every $10.00 spent on healthcare. More than 60 million visits to physicians are related to diabetes each year, and since 5.2 billion people are believed to be pre-diabetic or undiagnosed, these statistics are likely vastly minimized. Combined with an epidemic of obesity in both children and adults linked directly with diabetes, this disease poses a huge health challenge in North America. These numbers are truly staggering, especially considering that we now know that diabetes can be largely prevented – or at least more effectively managed – through dietary and lifestyle modifications.

Diabetes is a complicated disease, and you'll soon find that despite significant progress in our knowledge, there are still competing theories on causes, prevention, and even treatments. By having a better understanding of your own illness, you'll be equipped to make sound decisions in your own care and treatment. Preventive healthcare is essential in alleviating the health and financial costs associated with diabetes. This includes health education on diabetes prevention, effective and early diagnoses, and better management strategies to prevent diabetic complications. In addition to eliminating the suffering of diabetics, there is also a financial advantage to preventive treatments for diabetics. The American Diabetes Association claims that more money is currently spent on treating the chronic complications of diabetes than on standard diabetic care.

The good news is that the best prevention and treatment for diabetes is simply healthy living. In fact, many of the lifestyle and nutrition recommendations made in this book are also recommended for non-diabetics interested in disease prevention. This book, then, presents a number of opportunities. For the Type I diabetic, there is opportunity to get better control of blood sugar fluctuations and to prevent some of the long-term side effects of the disease. For the Type II diabetic, there is the possibility of managing and even reversing the condition with safe, natural therapies and lifestyle changes. And for the person with 'prediabetes' (hypoglycemia, hyperinsulinemia, and metabolic syndrome), there is the opportunity to prevent these conditions from resulting in progressively deteriorating health.

Naturopathic Medicine

Naturopathic medicine is a primary healthcare system based on the recognition that the human organism has an incredible self-healing capacity. Naturopathic medicine supports this self-healing potential using an eclectic mix of traditional therapies. The therapies used by naturopathic doctors include lifestyle counseling, clinical nutrition, botanical medicine, traditional Asian medicine, homeopathic medicine, acupuncture, physical therapies, and hydrotherapy. In their own way, each therapy supports the self-healing efforts of the body. The naturopathic physician selects appropriate modalities to use on a given individual patient based on traditional knowledge, modern research, and clinical experience. This practice of medicine is at once founded on the healing wisdom of many centuries and a distillation of current scientific research. This makes naturopathic medicine truly a mix of art and science.

Fundamental Principles of Naturopathic Medicine

✦ First, do no harm
✦ Support the self-healing potential of the body
✦ Address the fundamental causes of disease whenever possible
✦ Treat the whole person through individualized treatment
✦ Teach the principles of healthy living and preventive medicine

Naturopathic Medical Tradition

Naturopathic medicine developed from the ancient Greek medical tradition founded by Hippocrates, the father of Western medicine, based on the premise that the body has an inherent ability to heal, referred to in Latin as *Vis Medicatrix Naturae* (Healing Power of Nature). The human being was considered by the ancient Greek physicians to be a dynamic creation of body, mind, and spirit that was more than the sum of its parts.

These premises informed the founding of the naturopathic medical profession at the turn of the 20th century by a group of European and American physicians dedicated to the practice of botanical medicine, homeopathy, spinal manipulation, hydrotherapy, and nutritional therapy. Their vision was to educate a profession of medical practitioners who could synthesize the techniques, observations, and practices of many healing modalities. A name was needed for this profession: naturopathy, a neologism from the Latin for nature and the Greek for suffering, was chosen.

While naturopathic medicine thrived in the early 20th century under the influence of such notable physicians as Dr Benedict Lust and Dr Henry Lindlahr, the profession was eclipsed by surgical and pharmaceutical technological therapies. Naturopathic medical training was revived in the 1950s by Dr John Bastyr, after whom Bastyr University is named. Today there are six colleges of naturopathic medicine in North America: Bastyr University in Seattle, Washington; National College of Natural Medicine in Portland, Oregon; Southwest College of Naturopathic Medicine in Tempe, Arizona; Bridgeport University College of Naturopathic Medicine in Bridgeport, Connecticut; The Boucher Institute of Naturopathic Medicine in Vancouver, British Columbia; and The Canadian College of Naturopathic Medicine in Toronto, Ontario.

Together these institutions have an enrollment of more than 2,000 students. The curriculum is standardized and there is an accrediting body, The Council of Naturopathic Medical Education (CNME), which is recognized by the United States Department of Education. Graduates write international (Canada and the United States) licensing exams, which are known as the Naturopathic Physicians Licensing Exams (NPLEX). Upon passing NPLEX, they are eligible to practice in jurisdictions where naturopathic medicine is regulated.

Recently, naturopathic medicine has been given many alternative names – alternative, complementary, integrative, and holistic, to name a few. Regardless of the term used, one or more modalities of naturopathic medicine are now used by an estimated of 42% of the North American population. Visits to natural healthcare practitioners exceed visits to conventional primary care physicians by more than 200 million visits a year. North Americans spend more than an estimated $30 billion a year on these services. Many diabetes patients are seeking the advice of a naturopathic doctor for primary care or to complement the care already being received by conventional allopathic physicians.

Evidence-Based Medicine

A common misunderstanding about the practice of naturopathic medicine is that it is not 'scientific'. The naturopathic doctor is believed to be interested in diet and lifestyle factors only, not in the medical condition, and recommends treatments that have no evidence of efficacy. Nothing could be further from the truth.

For the patient's safety, the naturopathic doctor must establish a diagnosis based on medical history, physical examination, and standard laboratory tests. The diagnosis yields the information needed to select the appropriate naturopathic treatment. Once the etiology, pathogenesis, and pathophysiology of a condition are understood, the doctor can then recommend steps to restore normal physiological function. These therapeutic protocols are evidence-based in scientific literature and clinical practice, as the many references to peer-reviewed articles and refereed medical journals in this book testify.

Naturopathic Medicine Modalities

- Lifestyle Counseling
- Clinical Nutrition
- Botanical Medicine
- Traditional Asian Medicine (Chinese and Ayurvedic)
- Homeopathic Medicine
- Physical Therapies
- Hydrotherapy

Holistic Integrative Perspective

Naturopathic medicine approaches the patient from a holistic perspective. The role of the naturopathic physician is to support the self-healing ability of the whole being, in contrast to the symptom management we see in conventional surgical and pharmaceutical medicine, where each organ in the body has its own specialist.

The fundamental difference between scientific reductionistic medicine and holistic naturopathic medicine is the focus. Holistic medicine looks at the body as a whole because something is lost when looking at the human being as a collection of organs functioning independently. Holistic medicine is interested in understanding how, when one system is not working properly, it causes other problems in the body. There is a myriad of possible interactions within the human body. The physician must consider the 'trees' and the 'forest' at the same time.

Thus, a successful treatment for an endocrine illness, such as endometriosis, must consider not only the reproductive tract, but also the liver because it functions in the degradation of the hormone produced in the reproductive tract. Someone who treats osteoporosis should consider all the organs involved in calcium metabolism – the skin, liver, kidney, thyroid, parathyroid, and gastrointestinal tract. By supporting the health of the organs not only will the osteoporosis improve, but also many other health complaints will often improve as well. The health of the individual may improve to the extent that other potential diseases are prevented.

Another example is allergies. We do not develop allergies simply because we are deficient in antihistamines. We develop allergies for a host of reasons. Perhaps it is due to omega-3 oil deficiency in the mast cell membranes. Maybe the liver is not able to detoxify foreign substances properly, irritating the immune system. A dysbiosis in the intestinal tract may be irritating the gastrointestinal lymphoid tissue. Therefore, a successful treatment for allergies may involve treating the liver, improving digestion, and balancing the immune system.

Holistic remedies are designed to re-establish balance in the body. This is achieved by a synergy of ingredients acting broadly throughout the organism, guiding it gently (and often slowly) back to equilibrium. In contrast, contemporary therapeutic thinking often considers only rapid and intensive effects on isolated parameters. These effects are often compared to reference drugs that are isolated substances designed for a single effect. No drug ever has a single effect, as evidenced by the long list of side effects of most pharmaceutical medications. Herbal medicines are often considered worthy of use in the West only when they compare favorably to such reference drugs. Yet herbal medicines by their very nature often work very differently than their pharmaceutical counterparts. Herbal medicines have been documented to work in ways similar to pharmaceutical drugs at times, but also as nutritive agents that support new healthy tissue growth, as anti-oxidants that prevent tissue damage, and as tonics that support glandular function by providing precursor molecules, to name a few. Hence, they are well suited to a holistic medical approach, but difficult to study in randomized controlled trials that are designed to investigate the activity of an isolated active ingredient in a limited time frame.

Holistic concepts may actually help explain the therapeutic variability always seen in human clinical trials of both herbs and pharmaceutical medications. Contemporary medicine focuses on the diagnosis of disease, seeking medicines that chemically counter the pathologic results of the condition. Clinical trials of such medicines are conducted on large groups of people lumped together by the fact that they all suffer from the same diagnosis. We have already seen with the above examples, such as the possible causes of allergies, why this may be a problem. No investigation is made into the cause of the disease, only its manifestations. Success in these trials is measured by how well the medicine is seen to counter the pathologic change or its symptoms, quickly and effectively, in a significant proportion of the studied population. Variability in results from person to person is usually considered to be due to such factors as individual variations in the number of receptor sites, enzyme systems, liver detoxification pathways, etc. Conventional Western medical reductionism and specialization may be hindering our ability to understand the use of herbal medicines as agents whose clinical effects demonstrate their ability to re-establish health.

From the holistic viewpoint, there are no disease entities, only individuals suffering the results of an imbalance of ordering principles. The same disease, such as allergies, could result from any number of causes. Treatment would be very different in each case, and a medication that would be effective at curing the disease in all patients is inconceivable. All that could be hoped for (and this is often the case in modern Western pharmaceutical medicine) is to control the symptoms. Thus, the antihistamine is considered efficacious for allergies, yet side effects are common, and there is no mitigation in the disease state, as evidenced by the fact that the medication must be consumed regularly and indefinitely.

Traditional Chinese medicine, Indian (Ayurvedic) medicine, and the Eclectic tradition of Western herbalism have classified disease in ways that are very different from Western conventional medicine, based on seeing patients as individuals, each with a unique manifestation of a disease state. Many of the drugs of the modern pharmaceutical compendiums were derived from medicines used by these ancestors. However, by isolating and concentrating ingredients, or making molecular changes to naturally derived medicines to ensure patent rights, the synergy of multiple ingredients acting in concert may be lost – and the side effects and toxicities of modern pharmaceuticals may be gained.

This is not to say there is not a time and a place for modern pharmaceutical interventions; however, it is time for these allopathic approaches to share the stage with naturopathic approaches.

Naturopathic Therapies

This book focuses on lifestyle and nutritional choices, as well as botanical medicines, traditional Asian medicines, and physical therapies, that can reduce the risk of developing diabetes, reduce the complications of diabetes, and, in some cases, even reverse diabetes. Naturopathic medicine is particularly well-suited to these tasks.

Lifestyle Counseling

If you were to attempt to create as much diabetes as possible within a given society, the prescription would likely look very similar to the way North Americans currently live. For instance, by examining the epidemiological evidence, you would find that diabetes (Type II) increases with lack of exercise, high stress levels, poor nutrition, overweight, and obesity. According to the Center for Disease Control, more than one half of the American adult population does not get enough exercise. The rate of obesity in North America continues to increase, which, in turn, increases the risk of diabetes by an astounding factor of 20 times.

Naturopathic doctors are well aware of these lifestyle effects and are eager to educate, motivate, and support people who wish to prevent diabetes or are being treated for diabetes. Healthy lifestyle can go a long way toward the maintenance of healthy blood sugar levels. Combining a healthy lifestyle with proper diet, nutritional supplements, and herbs is a powerful combination for diabetes treatment and prevention.

Clinical Nutrition

Some foods have been shown to promote the development of diabetes, while other foods have been shown to prevent and mitigate diabetes. Naturopathic doctors are well versed in the use of clinical nutrition, which means designing a specific dietary regime for the individual patient. Naturopathic approaches can also be very effective for the individual who recognizes a need to lose weight as part of an overall health improvement plan.

Changes in dietary habits can have a remarkable effect on diabetes, with many diagnosed diabetics able to control their disease with diet and lifestyle changes alone. In fact, these are the recommended first-line approaches to managing Type II diabetes. However, even the best foods may be deficient in some nutrients, and some people suffering from conditions like diabetes may require higher levels of nutrients to regain and maintain good health. Nutritional supplements may be required in these cases to prevent deficiencies and to treat disease conditions.

Botanical Medicine

Many traditional herbal medicines have demonstrated effectiveness for preventing and treating Type II diabetes. In fact, herbal medicines have been used for thousands of years in practically every traditional culture for this purpose. Herbal medicines support blood sugar control holistically by supporting the organs that regulate blood sugar. Many herbs, when taken with a meal, have also been shown to slow the glycemic response. Certain herbs have also been shown to increase antioxidant levels in the body, which is of great interest to diabetes, since increasing antioxidant levels can be of benefit in treating and preventing the complications of diabetes, such as retinopathy, neuropathy, and nephropathy.

Traditional Asian Medicine

Diabetes has been a medical problem since antiquity. Although modern Western medicine and traditional Asian medicine (TAM) share the same treatment goals of reducing symptoms and preventing complications, their approaches to conceptualizing, diagnosing, and treating diabetes are very different. The most commonly employed therapeutic methods in TAM include acupuncture/moxibustion, herbal medicine, diet therapy, and mind/body exercises (such as Qigong and Tai Chi).

The *Huang Di Nei Jing* (*Yellow Emperor's Inner Classic*), which dates from the Han Dynasty (206 B.C.–220 A.D.), listed 13 herbal formulations for the treatment of Xiao-ke (wasting and thirsting disease). A number of these traditional herbs, including *Panax ginseng*, *Momodica charantia* (balsam pear), *Lagenaria siceraria* (bottle gourd), and *Psidium gnajava*, have been shown in modern research to reduce blood glucose levels. Acupuncture has also been shown in clinical and experimental studies to have a beneficial effect by lowering serum glucose levels, and in the treatment of diabetic peripheral neuropathy, one of the most common complications of diabetes.

Physical Therapies

High glucose levels in the blood are known to accelerate the aging process. Excess glucose binds to important proteins in the body in a process known as glycation. This process causes important proteins in the body to be damaged, including the proteins found in connective tissue, such as in the joints. This can lead to premature loss of function and increased stiffness. Physical therapies can counter this tendency by promoting flexibility, reducing pain without medications, and improving circulation and nerve function.

Complementary Approach

This book is a humble attempt to examine diabetes from a holistic perspective and to demonstrate that natural medicine has an integral and valuable role in promoting the health and balance of the endocrine system. At the same time that we encourage the investigation of alternative naturopathic therapies for preventing, treating, and reversing diabetes, we support the ongoing dialog concerning the integration of naturopathic alternative and allopathic conventional medicine in a complementary practice. The well-being of the patient is foremost in such a complementary approach, with the politics of naturopathic and allopathic advocates put aside. With the support of the healthcare consuming public, governments must play a role in ensuring that genuine progress is made in promoting novel ways to blend alternative medicine and modern science for the promotion of health. This is especially important in a time of demographic shift to a more elderly population, rising rates of chronic disease, including diabetes, and the strain placed on the availability and cost of healthcare services. May we all better understand the art of medicine, the science of the human organism, and the need for compassion and understanding.

The intention of this book is to empower diabetics, your families, and your practitioners by giving you the information you need to make informed decisions on your treatment while incorporating healthy changes into your daily routine. As diabetes affects more and more people, the only way to halt the spread of this epidemic is to take control of our own health. Making changes in the way we live our lives today will have a definite impact on our future, individually and collectively.

In this book, you will find information to help you better understand the physiological causes of diabetes mellitus and its various associated disorders, as well as proven and practical ways to prevent and manage its complications. Clinical trials are included to demonstrate the potential for both nutraceutical and botanical medicine in diabetes treatment. New areas of research and the threat to populations deemed particularly high-risk for developing diabetes are also discussed. By integrating technical information, scientific studies, and realistic suggestions, the information is accessible no matter your level of knowledge. If you have been recently diagnosed with diabetes and are feeling confused, simply skip to the sections that interest you or of most immediate benefit to you. You can always return to this book later when you have more of a grasp on your diabetes.

A diagnosis of diabetes doesn't need to discourage or isolate you if you view it as an occasion to make positive changes for your own health and the health of your family and friends. We trust this book can help you take the first steps.

Dr Alexander McLellan, ND
Dr Michaël Friedman, ND

(1) DIABETES BASICS

Diabetes is a chronic disorder affecting the metabolism of carbohydrates, fats, and proteins. Simply put, it is a condition characterized by an elevated blood glucose level after fasting for 24 hours. Ideally, the body would respond quickly and efficiently enough to a rise in blood glucose levels by secreting and utilizing insulin, the hormone responsible for increasing the rate at which cells absorb glucose. In diabetics, this control mechanism is faulty, and blood glucose levels remain elevated.

Diabetes is the main disease in a collection of disorders that affect our metabolism and blood glucose levels. Because diabetes is a metabolic disease that is affected by such menial daily activities as eating, drinking, exercising, and even relaxing, it is crucial to identify it early. Some early signs of the potential development of diabetes include hypoglycemic symptoms (when blood sugar drops quickly, resulting in shakiness and irritability) and metabolic syndrome X (a grouping of symptoms that include elevated cholesterol levels and high blood pressure). By understanding the physiology of diabetes and these potentially prediabetic conditions, you will be better equipped to seek medical guidance for any symptoms you experience. You will also be better able to make decisions on your treatment options.

Diabetes and Prediabetic Conditions

Type I Diabetes Mellitus: DMI usually begins in childhood and is due to insufficient insulin production by the pancreas. The cause is viral or autoimmune disease. Insulin allows glucose to travel from the blood into the cells, where it can be metabolized. When there isn't enough insulin, blood glucose levels become elevated.

Type II Diabetes Mellitus: DMII usually begins in adulthood and is often due to insulin resistance or improper response of insulin receptors to the insulin produced by the pancreas.

Hypoglycemia: The symptoms of hypoglycemia come on when blood sugar levels drop too low. Symptoms go away after eating, when blood sugar levels return to normal. The diagnosis of hypoglycemia is usually based on symptoms because blood sugar levels are only low at the time patients are experiencing symptoms.

Hyperinsulinemia: This condition is often a precursor to Type II diabetes. Patients can develop elevated insulin levels before they develop elevated blood glucose levels. The pancreas makes and secretes excessive amounts of insulin, presumably in an effort to compensate for insulin resistance.

Syndrome X: This syndrome refers to a metabolic syndrome of hyperinsulinemia that is associated with high blood pressure, high triglyceride levels, and low HDL levels. Predisposing factors include a family history of Type II diabetes, a diet high in carbohydrates, and a sedentary lifestyle. Truncal obesity, fatty liver, difficulty losing weight, and hypoglycemia often accompany this condition.

Type I Diabetes

In Type I insulin-dependent diabetes mellitus (IDDM), the beta cells of the pancreas fail to produce sufficient amounts of insulin to regulate blood sugar levels. Type I diabetes is called insulin dependent diabetes mellitus because it is characterized by the body's insufficient manufacture of insulin, resulting in excessively high blood glucose levels. In a healthy non-diabetic person, beta cells in the pancreatic islets are responsible for producing insulin, a hormone that allows glucose to be transported across cell membranes so that it can be used for energy. When these beta cells are destroyed, the result is insufficient insulin production by the pancreas. When there isn't enough insulin, blood glucose levels can become dangerously elevated.

The primary step in the development of diabetes mellitus is the activation of T lymphocytes, cells involved in the body's immunity against foreign invaders and especially against viral infections. It is believed that in Type I diabetes, T lymphocytes develop that target specific antigens present on the pancreatic beta cells. The antigen may be something seemingly harmless, but the immune system reacts forcefully by orchestrating a slow destruction of the beta cells.

This type of diabetes is usually associated with an early onset and represents only about 10% of diabetics. It is most often diagnosed in children and adolescents, but can occur at any stage of life. Although Type I diabetes can occur at any time, it usually develops before 30 years of age. Patients tend to be thin because the lack of insulin prevents most of the cells of the body from accessing the glucose fuel in the blood.

Type I diabetics are also prone to developing diabetic ketoacidosis, a condition which results from an excess breakdown of fat for energy. Ketones, byproducts of the breakdown of fats for energy, build up in the blood, and, if left unchecked, can produce a fruity smelling breath and impair judgment. Severe ketoacidosis is a medical emergency because it can render a person unconscious and can be fatal.

The other serious condition that Type I diabetics can experience is hypoglycemic coma. In this case, instead of excess glucose in the blood, the blood sugar drops excessively. This is typically due to excessive insulin injections.

Usually Type I diabetes requires routine treatments with exogenous insulin and close monitoring of blood glucose levels throughout your life.

Causes of IDDM

IDDM is an autoimmune condition, in which the immune system becomes confused and produces antibodies to attack the body's own tissues, in this case resulting in pancreatic destruction. Three quarters of Type I diabetics have antibodies present, and it is thought that they are produced in response to some foreign irritant. Although the definitive cause of diabetes remains elusive, there are a number of scientifically supported theories on the cause of beta cell destruction, discussed below.

Genetics

Traditionally, it was thought that Type I diabetes was caused by a genetic factor that resulted in the destruction of the beta cells, but this thesis has been increasingly discredited in more recent studies. Although genetic factors may increase our susceptibility to developing diabetes, they alone account for as little as 5% to 10% of cases of IDDM.

Viral Infections

Infections, particularly in childhood, seem to be linked to the development of diabetes mellitus. This connection was first reported in a Scandinavian study when two children developed diabetes mellitus after infection from the mumps. Another study conducted in London over a 10-year period tracked the seasonal incidence of the onset of Type I diabetes. In this study, virtually all cases of Type I diabetes developed in the fall and winter, the highest level being in October. This typically corresponds to periods of increased frequency of viral infections. Onset peaked at ages 5 and 11 years, which epidemiologists attribute to the time children undergo radical environmental changes as they move from home to school and are exposed to a high number of viruses. Suspected viral triggers for Type I diabetes include coxsackie b4 virus, mumps, and other as yet unidentified viruses.

Cow's Milk

Although not definitively conclusive, there is some evidence of a causal connection between exposure to cow's milk in infancy and the subsequent development of IDDM. *The New England Journal of Medicine* has reported that bovine serum albumin, or BSA, triggers an autoimmune response in genetically-susceptible children. Instead of just attacking BSA, the immune system begins to attack proteins on the surface of beta cells that are structurally similar to BSA, destroying the pancreas in the process.

Conversely, human breast milk may offer protection from diabetes. One study of 803 children up to 15 years of age in Sweden and Lithuania found that exclusive breast-feeding in infancy was correlated with a lower risk of developing IDDM. Protection was also associated with the delayed introduction of solid foods and cow's milk. Another study reported in *Pediatrics Diabetes* suggested that insulin, found in substantial concentrations in human milk but not in infant formulas, could prevent the development of diabetes.

Hyperglycemia Toxicity

Beta cell death resulting from hyperglycemia in diabetes Type II can cause insulin dependent diabetes in some cases. Hyperglycemia causes pancreatic beta cell damage in itself. From preliminary animal studies, it appears that beta cells fail to respond appropriately to glucose when glucose levels are kept above 120 mg/dl. By this mechanism, uncontrolled Type II diabetes can eventually turn into Type I. This is another example of how a pathology (hyperglycemia) can actually reinforce the illness itself by destroying the cells that counteract hyperglycemia. It is interesting to note that illnesses can often create feedback loops that are self-perpetuating.

The fasting glucose homeostasis is controlled by a balance between glucose utilization by peripheral tissues and hepatic glucose production. Non-diabetics are able to have fasting insulin levels that are sufficient to suppress hepatic gluconeogenesis through the production of glucagon. But insulin resistance and insulin deficiency found in Type I diabetes have no effective feedback loop for gluconeogenesis, and thus the liver will contribute to hyperglycemia.

Type II Diabetes

The more prevalent type of diabetes is referred to as Type II or non-insulin-dependent diabetes mellitus (NIDDM). In the United States, about 5.2% of the population (13 million people) has diabetes; 90% of these cases are non-insulin dependent diabetes (NIDDM). Of these

Characteristics of Type I and Type II Diabetes		
Characteristic	*Type I*	*Type II*
Prevalence (U.S.A.)	1.3 million (10%)	11.7 million (90%)
Onset	Childhood	Insidious onset: usually 40 + years old
Symptoms	Polyuria, polydipsia, weight loss, fatigue, and mycotic infections, diabetic ketoacidosis, nausea, vomiting, abdominal pain, dehydration, hypotension	Same symptoms though ketoacidosis is rare. History of hypertension and dyslipidemias.
Causes	Autoimmune: genetics, viral infection, cow's milk Hyperglycemia toxicity	Diet: low fiber, high refined sugar Obesity Glucose oxidation
Body Type	Thin	Obese
Insulin	Low insulin: body can't make insulin.	Insulin resistance: cells are desensitized to insulin
Complications	Cardiovascular disease, neuropathy, nephropathy, cataracts, and retinal disease.	Same. May be the first signs of disease.

people, 90% can be classified as overweight or obese. Although this type of diabetes used to occur mostly in adults over 40 years of age, it is now being diagnosed in children as young as 10 years of age.

In NIDDM, insulin levels are typically elevated, indicating that the beta cells are functioning to produce what should be sufficient amounts of insulin, but a number of factors have caused the body's cells to lose sensitivity to the hormone. Thus, blood sugar levels remain dangerously elevated.

Unlike Type I diabetes, which always results in a deficiency in insulin, there are a number of ways in which Type II diabetes manifests. In some patients, there is a decreased production of insulin, but this is not always the case. NIDDM with insulin resistance occurs when the body produces insulin, but becomes desensitized to it and thus fails to react. Some Type II patients may even have increased insulin production to compensate for this resistance.

Hyperinsulinemia is a frequently overlooked precursor to NIDDM, in which excessive secretions of insulin causes a condition similar to mild insulin shock, but more chronic in nature.

Causes of NIDDM

There are many proposed explanations of the mechanisms involved in the development of NIDDM. This type of diabetes is consistently associated with a diet high in refined foods, obesity, and a sedentary lifestyle.

Diet

A low-fiber diet that is high in refined sugars and fats can contribute to the development of reactive hypoglycemia. Refined carbohydrates cause a rapid rise in blood sugar levels, and the resulting insulin surges may lead to hypoglycemia. In response, the adrenal glands secrete epinephrine, cortisol, and other stress hormones to return blood sugar levels back to normal. If patients continually assault their bodies with this type of refined diet, it may result in both pancreatic and adrenal exhaustion.

Obesity

Obesity is a significant risk factor for developing NIDDM. Type II patients comprise about 90% of all diabetics, and of these, the vast majority are overweight or obese. In fact, excess weight is the primary predictor of Type II diabetes. A 2001 American random telephone survey of nearly 200,000 subjects concluded that being overweight or obese was significantly associated with diabetes, among other diseases. When compared with normal-weight subjects, those with a body mass index (BMI) of 40 or higher were more than seven times more likely to have been diagnosed with diabetes.

Research indicates that obesity often precedes the oversecretion of insulin. Oversecretion of insulin leads to resistance of the cells to the actions of insulin. This results in increased production of insulin by the pancreas and an ensuing vicious cycle that results in hyperinsulinemia, or high insulin levels in the blood. This can start early in life. Obesity in childhood and adolescence is significantly associated with insulin resistance, dyslipidemia, and elevated blood pressure in young adulthood. The good news, however, is that weight loss by obese young people has been shown to result in a decrease in insulin concentration and improvement in insulin sensitivity. On the basis of our current knowledge, it is, therefore, reasonable to suggest that lifestyle modification and weight control reduces the risk of developing Type II diabetes mellitus later in life.

Glucose Oxidation

Another postulated mechanism of how obesity contributes to the development of NIDDM is via a problem with the metabolism of glucose at the cellular level. Glucose metabolism is regulated by an enzyme known as pyruvate-dehydrogenase (PDH), and inhibited by isomers of another enzyme, pyruvate-dehydrogenase kinase (PDK). Increased levels of PDK may cause insulin resistance and increased fatty acid oxidation in NIDDM patients. Recent studies have found that obesity can cause increased levels of PDK, which impairs glucose oxidation and thus results in increased fatty acid oxidation.

Fortunately, this type of diabetes often responds exceptionally well to changes in diet, and in a large number of people can be prevented and even reversed entirely by making healthful lifestyle modifications.

Hepatic Insulin Sensitizing Substance

Glucose homeostasis is regulated both by the pancreas and the counter-regulatory responses of the adrenal gland and liver. The hormones involved include glucagon, catecholamines, growth hormone, and cortisol. The role of the liver in NIDDM has been demonstrated in both animal and human studies. Receptors on hepatic parasympathetic nerves release nitric oxide, which causes the release of hepatic insulin sensitizing substance (HISS). HISS sensitizes skeletal muscle to absorb insulin. Animal studies have shown that the blockade of nitric oxide release causes a secondary blockade of HISS, which results in insulin resistance.

Low Birth Weight

Low birth weight and poor infant nutrition create lifelong health risks and are contributing factors in the development of NIDDM. Inadequate calories during fetal growth may be diverted to the development of organs other than the pancreas, or may encourage genes to become thriftier in maximizing available calories. This is problematic in later periods of caloric abundance. The abnormal development of pancreas and adipose tissues resulting from decreased fetal nutrition thus contributes to hyperglycemia in adulthood.

Key Terms

Blood sugar: A measure of the amount of glucose in the blood. Control of blood glucose is the most vital component of diabetes management.

Glucagon: A hormone secreted by the pancreas, which increases the concentration of glucose in the blood.

Glycogen: A storage form of carbohydrate, which the body can convert to back to glucose when needed.

Insulin: A hormone secreted by the pancreas (beta cells), which is essential for the proper metabolism of glucose.

Insulin resistance: A cellular blunting of the effects of insulin on the ability to metabolize glucose.

Hormonal Interactions

Endocrine tissue found in the pancreatic islets forms the basis of blood sugar control. This tissue secretes hormones that serve to either increase or decrease blood sugar, maintaining a delicate energy balance within the body. These hormones are called glucagon and insulin.

This interaction between our hormones is complicated. A delicate balance of input versus output must be maintained. Type I diabetics are missing a key player in this interaction. Without adequate insulin, the blood glucose level remains elevated. In addition, instead of responding to high blood sugar levels, glucagon will continue to try to increase blood sugar. This is because insulin levels control glucagon release. If insulin levels remain low even when blood sugar is high, glucagon will continue to try to raise blood glucose levels.

In Type II diabetes, the pancreas is trying to communicate with the cells, but the cells are no longer sensitive to the message. For this reason, Type II diabetes is also called insulin resistance. Typically, this lack of sensitivity to insulin by the cells is the result of years of high levels of simple carbohydrate consumption combined with a sedentary lifestyle. This causes the pancreas to produce excess amounts of insulin, but eventually the cells become 'resistant' to its effects, and the blood glucose rises. In essence, the pancreatic release of insulin resembles a 'crying wolf' effect, but the cells of the body are no longer listening, even though the situation has become an emergency because the blood glucose is elevated.

Stress hormone release exacerbates problems with blood glucose control. This is true for endogenous stress hormones (those released by the body's own glands, such as cortisol and epinephrine) or exogenous stress hormones (those taken as medication, such as corticosteroids). Thus, for both types of diabetics, stress can at minimum make short-term control of blood sugar more challenging, but in the long term can be quite dangerous by contributing to the chronic complications that diabetics tend to develop.

The goal of diabetic therapy is to restore efficient communication between these systems. This can be achieved in some milder cases by strengthening the pancreas to produce more insulin or, more typically, by taking exogenous doses of insulin.

Glucagon and Glycogen

Pancreatic Alpha (A) cells in the periphery of the pancreas islet tissue secrete glucagon, a polypeptide hormone that increases blood sugar. When extra energy is consumed, it is stored as glycogen in the liver and muscles. Glycogen is essentially many glucose molecules bound together for storage. Glucagon works by binding to glycogen receptors on the liver and inducing the enzymatic breakdown of glycogen to glucose. Simply put, glucagon signals the liver to release stored glucose back into the bloodstream.

Glucagon also functions in the formation of glucose from amino acids in the liver through a process called gluconeogenesis. This allows some of the excess protein consumed in the diet to be shunted into energy production.

Insulin

Adjacent to the alpha cells in the pancreas are the beta cells. They constitute 70% of the islet cells and function to lower blood sugar with the secretion of insulin. Insulin is essential for the uptake of glucose from the blood into the majority of the body's cells. Insulin manufacture and sensitivity plays the major role in diabetes. In Type I diabetes, beta cells are destroyed through what is thought to be an autoimmune response, resulting in insufficient insulin secretion. In Type II diabetes, there is usually a loss of sensitivity to insulin at the cellular level, compromising the cell's ability to utilize glucose. In both Type I and Type II diabetes, glucose can no longer get from the blood into the cell efficiently, and levels of glucose in the blood rise.

Virtually all cells use insulin in order to absorb glucose, except for the tissues found in the retina of the eye, nerves, and kidneys. Insulin allows sugar to enter the cells by increasing the number of proteins that transport glucose across cell membranes, and by activating existing transport proteins. Insulin also increases the synthesis of glycogen from glucose in liver cells. In the tissues, where insulin is not required for the entry of glucose into the cell, the excess glucose that freely enters the cells is broken down into sugar alcohols (polyols). When in excess, these sugar alcohols contribute to the secondary complications of diabetes found in the retinas, nerves, and kidneys of diabetics.

The effects of insulin are numerous, including mediating storage of carbohydrates, fats, and proteins. Insulin also facilitates cellular growth and enhances liver, adipose, and muscle metabolism. Hence, while those with Type I diabetes tend to lose weight due to a lack of insulin, those with Type II are typically overweight due to the effects of excess insulin production. Excess insulin production tends to deposit weight around the trunk (producing the so called 'spare tire'), which is a risk factor for a number of chronic diseases, including cardiovascular disease.

DHEA and Cortisol

Imbalances of the hormones DHEA and cortisol influence blood sugar control and are contributing factors to the development of diabetes. In general, insulin resistance is associated with low DHEA levels, especially in men. Insulin resistance in women is usually associated with adrenal hypersecretion and polycystic ovary syndrome. High levels of DHEA and cortisol are typical of this subset of patients.

Cortisol is released in response to physical, metabolic, or psychological stress and raises blood sugar by stimulating gluconeogenesis in hepatic and skeletal muscle tissues. Thus, chronically high levels contribute to insulin resistance, abdominal fat deposits (apple-shaped obesity), and lipid abnormalities – the constellation of imbalances associated with metabolic syndrome X.

DHEA is a precursor of testosterone and estrogen synthesis. DHEA is also an important hormone with its own receptors and physiological properties. DHEA stimulates increased lean muscle mass and reduced abdominal fat. It also appears to play an important role in glucose regulation. Most importantly, experimental studies show that DHEA administration increases insulin sensitivity. DHEA levels are typically higher in men. High levels in women may be associated with hirsutism and insulin resistance.

Insulin Like Growth Factor (IGF-I)

Produced in the liver in response to growth hormone stimulus, IGF-1 (insulin like growth factor 1) plays an important role in regulating glucose metabolism. IGF-1 helps to increase insulin sensitivity. It also works in the body to increase lean muscle mass, enhance fat metabolism, and improve cardiovascular function. Research studies indicate that IGF-1 cuts the rate of diabetes by nearly 50% in laboratory animals by protecting pancreatic beta cells from autoimmune destruction. In addition, low levels of IGF-1 have been associated with atherosclerosis, aging, obesity, and the development of diabetic neuropathy.

Hormonal Conversations

One way to understand the relationship between blood sugar metabolism and diabetes is to imagine a daily 'conversation' between our hormones. Each and every day, a balancing act is carried out within our endocrine system. The central players are:

Pancreas: gland that contains the pancreatic islets, tissue responsible for producing and secreting insulin and glucagon.

Adrenal glands: glands that secrete stress hormones, including cortisol and epinephrine.

Glucagon: a pancreatic hormone that releases stored glycogen from the muscles and liver back into the blood.

Insulin: a pancreatic hormone that allows glucose to be moved across cell membranes for energy production.

Cortisol: an adrenal gland hormone released when stress is chronic and long-term.

Epinephrine: an adrenal gland hormone also known as adrenaline that is released during a 'fight or flight' response.

Act 1, Scene 1: In the early morning while you're still sleeping, your blood glucose level hovers near 70 mg/dl (4 mmol/L). When your alarm clock sounds, your blood sugar rises in response to the secretion of cortisol and epinephrine.

Act 1, Scene 2: When you arrive at work, your boss blames you for someone else's mistake. You become agitated and frustrated, and your blood sugar increases again as stress hormones surge from your adrenal glands. You sit down at your desk and play your favorite relaxation tape. As you calm down, your stress hormone levels decrease, reducing your blood sugar.

Act 2, Scene 1: By lunchtime, your blood sugar has dropped again to about 50 mg/dl (2.8 mmol/L). You eat lunch and treat yourself to a scoop of ice cream for dessert. Your blood sugar rises to 100 mg/dl (5.6 mmol/L) and your pancreas responds by secreting insulin. This pushes the glucose into your cells, returning your blood sugar levels to a normal range.

Act 2, Scene 2: After work, you spring to your bus stop to catch an early bus. Glucagon enables the quick release of stored glycogen to fuel your energy burst. Once you arrive home, your hormones continue their 'conversation' as you relax, exercise, eat, and prepare for bed. Tomorrow morning, their interaction will continue to monitor your blood sugar as it rises and falls while you carry on with your daily life. In fact, these interactions between hormones are taking place every minute of every hour of your life.

Coda: People with diabetes mellitus are missing something in their hormonal conversation. Their ability to produce or use insulin is diminished. The hormones that tell the body to increase the blood sugar may be working, but the insulin that brings blood sugar down does not respond. Glucagon responds to low insulin levels, but it does not respond to low blood sugar levels. This is why the one-way conversation of the counter regulatory hormones can be quite dangerous in a diabetic. Glucagon will keep on increasing blood sugar by responding to low insulin levels, rather than responding to the high blood sugar levels, which can eventually lead to a coma.

Diabetic Therapy: The goal of diabetic therapy is to restore the communication in the body between these systems. This can be achieved by strengthening the pancreas to produce more insulin, by restoring peripheral metabolism of insulin, or by taking exogenous insulin.

Prediabetic Conditions

Although much of the existing literature on diabetes deals specifically with diabetes mellitus, it is important to recognize that there is a wide range of blood sugar disorders. Particularly in North America, diets high in refined carbohydrates, combined with inactive lifestyles, are contributing to growing numbers of people with insulin resistance, hypoglycemia, hyperinsulinemia, and syndrome X. This puts our population at risk for diabetic complications, cardiovascular disease, and other serious conditions.

Insulin Resistance and Hyperinsulinemia

Information on insulin resistance is of critical importance because the metabolic changes that precede the development of diabetes often occur 10 or more years before the disease actually manifests. Early recognition of insulin resistance can help prevent hyperinsulinemia, dyslipidemia, hormonal imbalances, increased mortality rates, and cardiac risk. Many people can develop some of the complications of diabetes, such as peripheral neuropathy, even before their blood glucose levels are consistently outside standard normal blood test ranges. Thus, part of early recognition of the potential for diabetes to develop includes monitoring for glucose levels in the 'high normal' range and looking for symptoms that may be related to diabetic complications.

Hypoglycemia

Hypoglycemia, or low blood sugar, occurs when blood glucose values are less than 50 mg/dl (2.8 mmol/L). The three essential aspects of hypoglycemia as described by Whipple's triad are: low plasma glucose, symptoms associated with hypoglycemia, and symptomatic resolution when blood sugar is returned back to normal. The diagnosis of hypoglycemia is usually based on symptoms because blood sugar levels are only low while patients are experiencing symptoms.

The adrenergic symptoms related to hypoglycemia are linked to catecholamine levels. These symptoms include diaphoresis (sweating), palpitations, apprehension, anxiety, headache, and weakness. The lack of blood sugar supply to the brain will cause neuroglycopenic symptoms and result in confusion, irritability, abnormal behavior, 'spaciness', and possibly even convulsions and coma.

Fasting Hypoglycemia

Severe fasting hypoglycemia usually indicates an organic cause. These include pancreatic disorders, liver disease, pituitary-adrenal disorders, CNS disease, non-pancreatic neoplasms, and idiopathic hypoglycemia of childhood.

Pseudohypoglycemia

Pseudohypoglycemia is a false positive laboratory reading of hypoglycemia that happens due to chronic leukemia, hemolytic anemia, or polycythemia. The mechanism for the false positive in leukemia is due to the glucose utilization by leucocytes in the blood sample after it has been drawn from the patient.

Reactive Hypoglycemia

Reactive hypoglycemia, also called postprandial hypoglycemia, is by far the most common form and tends to be misdiagnosed or overlooked. It results from the poor function of the organs that regulate blood sugar. Symptoms range from irritability when meals are missed to drastic mood swings, and their wide breadth may be confused with other disorders. It is associated with food cravings, particularly for sweets or carbohydrates, but once these foods are consumed, sluggishness occurs rather than satiation.

Syndrome X

Syndrome X refers to a metabolic syndrome of hyperinsulinemia that is associated with high blood pressure, high triglyceride levels, and low HDL ('good' cholesterol) levels. Predisposing factors include a family history of Type II diabetes, a diet high in carbohydrates, and a sedentary lifestyle. Truncal obesity, fatty liver, difficulty losing weight, and hypoglycemia often accompany this condition.

The symptoms of diabetes are broad and are often confused with other illnesses. The most recognizable symptoms are excessive thirst and urination as the kidneys attempt to flush the blood of excess glucose. Some patients experience 'spaciness', mild to severe depression, irritability, excessive sweating, confusion or incoherent speech, anxiety, headaches, convulsions, blurred vision, and bizarre behavior. Approximately half of all diabetics remain undiagnosed, so if you're experiencing a vague collection of symptoms similar to those listed here, it's important to discuss them with a healthcare provider.

Signs and Symptoms

Type I Diabetes

- Typical symptoms include polyuria, polydipsia, weight loss despite a normal or increased dietary intake, fatigue, and opportunistic infections, such as mycotic infections.
- Diabetic ketoacidosis may develop if DM type I is left untreated. Nausea, vomiting, abdominal pain, dehydration, hypotension, and even coma can result.

- Diabetes Type I increases risk of cardiovascular disease, neuropathy, nephropathy, cataracts, and retinal disease.

Type II Diabetes

- Typically, this condition comes on insidiously over several years. Symptoms can be similar to Type I, but without the propensity to ketoacidosis.
- Patients are usually over 30, overweight or obese, and may have a history of hypertension and dyslipidemias.
- Long-term complications are similar as those mentioned for Type I, although in this case, complications, such as neuropathy, mycotic infections, or eye disease, may be the first clue to a disease state.
- Family history of Type II diabetes.
- Diet high in refined carbohydrates, deficient in dietary fiber.
- Lack of physical exercise.
- Truncal obesity, hypertension, skin tags, cataracts, opportunistic infections.

Hypoglycemia

- Tired all the time
- Hungry between meals or at night
- Depressed
- Insomnia, awakening with inability to return to sleep
- Wake up after a few hours sleep
- Fearful (overwhelmed by people, places, or things)
- Can't decide easily
- Can't concentrate
- Poor memory
- Worry frequently
- Highly emotional
- Moody
- Cry easily, or feel like crying inside
- Fits of anger
- Magnify insignificant details (mountains out of molehills)
- Eat candy, cake; or drink soda pop
- Eat bread, pasta, potatoes, rice, or beans

- Consume alcohol
- Drink more than three cups of coffee or cola drinks daily
- Crave candy, soda, or coffee between meals or mid-afternoon
- Can't work well under pressure
- Headaches
- Sleepy during the day
- Sleepy or drowsy after meals
- Lack of energy
- Can't get started in the morning
- Stomach cramps or 'nervous stomach'
- Allergies: asthma, hay fever, skin rash, sinus trouble, etc.
- Fatigue relieved by eating
- Suicidal thought or tendencies; feeling of hopelessness
- Bored
- Bad dreams
- Irritable before meals
- Heart beats fast (palpitations)
- Get shaky inside when hungry
- Feel faint if meal is delayed
- Ulcers, gastritis, chronic indigestion, abdominal bloating
- Cold hands or feet
- Blurred vision
- Bleeding gums
- Dizziness, giddiness, or lightheadedness
- Aware of breathing heavily
- Bruise easily
- Reduced sex drive
- Poor coordination (drop or bump into things)
- Sweating excessively
- Unsocial or antisocial behavior
- Muscle twitching or cramps
- Skin aches or itches
- Phobias (excessive fear or some thing or situation)
- Hallucinations
- Convulsions
- Trembling (shaking) hands

Hyperinsulinemia

Many of these symptoms are also associated with hypoglycemia, or low blood sugar.

- Weight gain
- Cravings for sugar
- Intense hunger
- Weakness
- Need for frequent meals
- Poor concentration
- Emotional instability
- Memory loss
- Lack of focus
- Feelings of anxiety or panic
- Lack of motivation
- Fatigue

Syndrome X

- Syndrome X is a pre-diabetic condition resulting from insulin resistance without necessarily elevated blood glucose levels.
- Truncal obesity resistant to calorie restriction, elevated triglycerides, and low HDL cholesterol are common findings.
- Fatigue (especially after meals with a high glycemic index or load), skin tags, Dupuytren's contracture, Peyronie's disease, osteoarthritis, hypoglycemia, and sugar cravings may also be present.

Physical Exam

Screening for early signs and symptoms of diabetes, followed by regular physical examinations for those diagnosed, cannot be overemphasized. In fact, nearly 25% of diabetic diagnoses are made during a routine physical examination, according to the National Institutes of Health (NIH). In addition, nearly half of adults diagnosed with Type II diabetes indicated that they had no symptoms of the disease at the time they were diagnosed, and most people have had the disease an average of 10 years prior to diagnosis.

Based on these statistics, there are an estimated 10 million North Americans who have diabetes and have not yet been diagnosed. In addition, approximately 40% of American adults between the ages 40 and 74 (about 41 million people) have prediabetes, according to the NIH. Prediabetes places these individuals at an increased risk for developing cardiovascular disease and Type II diabetes. Prediabetes is defined as having an elevated glucose (blood sugar) level that is above normal, but not high enough to be considered diabetes.

A physical examination is, therefore, an important part of detecting prediabetes. Detection of prediabetes or metabolic syndrome X can provide important time and motivation to make dietary and lifestyle changes, which will delay or even prevent a future diabetes diagnosis. Even if a diagnosis of diabetes has been made, regular physical examinations help to minimize the risk of developing serious complications.

Physical Exam for Diabetes

* **Height and weight measurement:** Being overweight or obese is an important risk factor for Type II diabetes. Children and teens should have their height and weight compared to standards that are normal for their age groups.
* **Blood pressure:** BP tends to be elevated in metabolic syndrome and diabetes.
* **Dilated eye exam:** Typically done by an ophthalmologist, this test looks for changes in the small blood vessels at the back of the eye.
* **Skin examination:** For dry, scaly skin, poor wound healing, fungal infections.
* **Thyroid exam:** Thyroid dysfunction often co-exists with blood sugar irregularities.
* **Peripheral pulses:** Pulses in the wrists, foot, and groin help to detect peripheral occlusions, which are a complication of diabetes.
* **Foot exam:** For fungal infections, sores, etc. Seeing a podiatrist who treats diabetics may be indicated.
* **Neurological exam:** This includes pinprick and vibratory sensation in the extremities because peripheral neuropathy is a common complication of elevated blood glucose.

Laboratory Tests

* Oral glucose insulin tolerance test (GITT) is indicated if hyperinsulinemia is suspected.
* Fasting plasma glucose is the typical diagnostic test for diabetes mellitus.
* Hemoglobin A1c is a useful measure of average blood glucose over a 2- to 3-month time span.
* Serum lipids (triglycerides, LDL, HDL, total cholesterol), lipoprotein A, and homocysteine are useful to assess cardiovascular risk.
* Cortisol and DHEA tests to assess adrenal function because increased cortisol and decreased DHEA are typical in insulin resistance.

Laboratory Tests

Among the various laboratory tests for diabetes, the following three are most common.

Oral Glucose Tolerance Test

An oral glucose tolerance test can be used to confirm a diagnosis of diabetes. The subject fasts for a specific period, after which 75 g of anhydrous glucose dissolved in water is administered. However, rarely is this test necessary in clinical practice because the measurement of elevated fasting plasma glucose done on two separate days should suffice in the diagnosis of diabetes.

Fasting Glucose Levels

Fasting levels can be obtained after an 8-hour fasting period. In a healthy person, the level should be equal to or lower than 110 mg/dl (6.1 mmol/L). A higher result indicates impaired glucose homeostasis. Diabetes is diagnosed at a level equal to or greater than 126 mg/dl (7.0 mmol/L). If a blood sugar test is conducted at any time of the day, including after a meal, and the results are equal to or greater than 200 mg/dl (11.1 mmol/L), diabetes is indicated.

Fructosamine and Hemoglobin A1c

A comprehensive dysglycemic metabolic profile also includes fructosamine and hemoglobin A1c (HbA1c). Fructosamine is a good short-term indicator of average glucose levels (10-14 days). It is a measure of how glucose levels are affecting proteins in the blood. Fructosamine is a sensitive marker of a patient's recent glycemic control, allowing practitioners to monitor treatment effectiveness over a shorter intervention period. High fructosamine levels may also be an important warning signal for increased risk of cardiovascular disease and mortality. Some research has shown a 4.3-fold increase in cardiovascular related deaths for women with high fructosamine levels.

HbA1c measures longer-term blood glucose control over a period of 2 to 3 months. Also known as glycated hemoglobin, HbA1c measures the effects of glucose on red blood cells. Since red blood cells live for an average of 3 months, HbA1c levels reflect average blood glucose levels during a 3-month time period. Thus, HbA1c levels help assess how well an individual is controlling glucose levels on average. As with fructosamine, there is a correlation between HbA1c levels and coronary heart disease risk. Higher levels of HbA1c have also been associated with other debilitating complications of diabetes, such as erectile dysfunction, retinopathy, and neurological disease.

③ | DIABETES RISK FACTORS

Your inherited genetic code can influence your susceptibility to developing both types of diabetes. Type II diabetes, by far the most prevalent form of diabetes, is almost always associated with identifiable and preventable risk factors. Education and behavior modification is the key to managing these risks. Type II diabetes in North America is predominantly a lifestyle related disease, not a genetic one.

The presence of one or more risk factors in a given individual should not in any way be construed as a prediction that the development of diabetes is inevitable. Rather, risk factors are presented as motivators to action. Even Type I diabetes, for which the strongest genetic correlation exists (23% to 38% genetic predisposition, depending on the study) is not inevitable. Vitamin D, for example, has been shown to have the potential to prevent over 80% of Type I diabetes if given in infancy.

Genetics

If your parents or other family members have Type I diabetes, you should be particularly aware of its symptoms. Studies have shown that there is a 2.1% risk that a child of a diabetic mother will also develop diabetes, and a 6.1% risk if the child's father is diabetic. This is compared to a 0.4% risk in the general North American population.

Type II diabetes also tends to run in families. Medical researchers have been studying genetic factors that may contribute to the onset of Type II diabetes over many years. There is good evidence of genetic connections to NIDDM. A complex combination of many genes may increase a person's risk for developing diabetes as an adult. These include genes associated with beta cell function, liver function, and pancreatic response to blood glucose levels.

Environmental Factors

Monozygotic twins (with identical genetic codes) have a 50% chance of becoming diabetic if one of the twins has diabetes. This means that the development of Type I diabetes is not dictated solely by genetics, or we would expect all those with the exact same genetic code to develop diabetes. In fact, out of 100 people with Type I diabetes, 80 have no family members with the disease. Clearly, the disease develops (as is the case with many diseases) from a complex mix of inherited and environmental factors.

Type I Diabetes

Viral Infections

Infections may be the cause of Type I diabetes mellitus. It was first reported in a Scandinavian study that two children developed diabetes mellitus after the mumps. In a study done in London over a 10-year period, scientists tracked the seasonal incidence of the onset of diabetes Type I. Virtually all reported cases of Type I developed in the fall and winter, the highest level being in October.

Onset peaks at age 5 and 11, which epidemiologists attribute to the time children undergo radical environmental changes as they move from home to school, where they are exposed to a high number of viruses. Suspected triggers for Type I diabetes include coxsackie b4 virus, mumps, and other unidentified diabetagenic viruses. Some researchers think that the virus triggers an immune reaction against the islet cells or, in rare cases, directly infects and kills these cells.

Clinical Studies: Cow's Milk and Diabetes

Studies

Research published in *The New England Journal of Medicine* has linked bovine serum albumin (BSA) to an autoimmune response that triggers diabetes. Other research has examined the possible connection between an allergic response to milk and the eventual development of diabetes. One Finnish study of 1,198 children measured levels of antibodies in children exposed to cow's milk at varying ages. The researchers concluded that the earlier cow's milk was introduced, the higher the level of antibodies exhibited. Furthermore, increased consumption of dairy products and cow's milk was positively correlated with higher levels of antibodies. By comparing diabetic and non-diabetic siblings, the researchers were able to isolate a connection between high levels of IgA antibodies and the increased risk of type I diabetes. They concluded that early introduction and high consumption of cow's milk and dairy products during childhood led to an increased risk of developing IDDM because of the antibodies elicited.

Another study at the University of Colorado, School of Medicine, was able to differentiate between the affect of cow's milk exposure on subjects at low or high risk of developing diabetes. In order to do this, they isolated a molecular marker (HLA-DQB1) for diabetes, accounting for other factors, including genetic susceptibility. Their results indicated that early exposure to cow's milk did not pose a threat to subjects at low risk for developing diabetes. However, subjects with the molecular marker had a strong correlation between early exposure to both cow's milk and solid foods, and the eventual development of IDDM.

Researchers at McMaster University in Canada published a convincing critical review of literature pertaining to cow's milk exposure and its relation to diabetes in *Diabetes Care*. They found that IDDM was consistently correlated with early exposure to cow's milk and diminished breast-feeding. Their review concluded that the increased risk for IDDM may be 1.5 times higher for those children who were fed cow's milk before 4 months of age.

Recommendation

Given this information, it seems reasonable to encourage mothers to breast-feed their infants, if at all possible, to reduce the exposure to cow's milk in early life. Alternative 'milks' are also now widely available, including those made from soy, nuts, and rice, that may be suitable for children at risk for diabetes. Infant soy formulas may be a consideration for infants whose mothers are unable to breast-feed in order to reduce the risk of diabetes.

We recommend that, if possible, children be breast-fed exclusively for the first 6 months. Food introduction should focus on vegetables and fruits from age 6 months to 1 year. Only after 1 year of age should you consider introducing cow's milk and other foods that may induce allergy, such as gluten-containing grains. It is also important to maintain good digestive health in children by supplementing with the probiotics *Lactobacillus acidophilus* and *Bifidus*, especially during and after courses of antibiotics.

Cow's Milk

Other than viruses, foods have also been linked to Type I. Cow's milk ingested in the first 6 to 8 weeks of infancy has been speculated as causing an autoimmune response to the milk by a process called molecular mimicry. The body produces antibodies against an antigen, such as bovine albumin peptide in cow's milk, which mimics the pancreatic cells of the body. As a result, the white blood cells attack the pancreas. Review of the medical literature indicates that ingestion of cow's milk increases the risk of Type I diabetes by a factor of 1.5. Some doctors now recommend breast-feeding at-risk children and limiting their intake of cow's milk.

Type II Diabetes

According to the National Institutes of Health, the risk factors for developing Type II diabetes are:

- Advancing age
- Overweight
- Having a parent, brother, or sister with diabetes
- Family background that is Alaska Native, American Indian, African American, Hispanic/Latino American, Asian American, or Pacific Islander
- History of gestational diabetes, or having given birth to at least one baby weighing more than 9 pounds
- Blood pressure 140/90 mm Hg or higher

- Cholesterol levels not normal. HDL ('good') cholesterol is below 35 mg/dL, or triglyceride level is above 250 mg/dL.
- Inactive lifestyle and exercise fewer than three times a week
- Polycystic ovary syndrome, also called PCOS (women only)
- On previous testing, evidence of impaired glucose tolerance (IGT) or impaired fasting glucose (IFG) detected
- History of cardiovascular disease

The risk for developing Type II diabetes can be also be identified by a number of contributing factors:
- Greater than 120% desirable body weight
- Imbalances of DHEA, cortisol, and IGF-1
- Sedentary lifestyle
- High consumption of refined carbohydrates, including fast food and soft drinks
- Nitric oxide deficiency
- Delivering a baby weighing more than 9 pounds
- Gestational diabetes
- Low birth weight
- Immune deregulation
- Vitamin and mineral deficiencies

High-Risk Populations

Aboriginal Populations

Diabetes among aboriginal people was virtually unheard of in the 1940s, but today the risk of Type II diabetes among aboriginal populations in North America is estimated at three to five times higher than for non-natives. And the number of cases of diabetes is expected to triple over the next 20 years. Diet, lack of exercise, genetics, and stress contribute to the problem, as does lack of access to fresh food in aboriginal communities, especially in the North.

In terms of diet, aboriginal people have undergone a rapid transition from a hunter-gatherer diet (low carbohydrate) to a diet high in refined carbohydrates. At the same time, a hunter-gatherer genetic profile (sometimes called 'thrifty genes') promotes fat storage and excess weight for utilization during times of scarcity. Since, in modern society, scarcity is rare for the majority, this thrifty genetic makeup increases the risk of obesity and diabetes.

Also of note is that foods high in trans fats, high in sugar, high in salt, and high in chemical preservatives are very inexpensive and have a long shelf life, often making them more affordable and more available to First Nations peoples in remote locations. At the same time, modern convenience has reduced the need to expend high amounts of calories to survive.

It has been estimated that an average hunter/gatherer existence requires the expenditure of 5000-6000 calories per day, whereas 2000-3000 calories per day of energy expenditure is more typical of an industrialized society with a predominance of activities requiring little physical exertion. In addition, traditional native food sources have been shown to be much more nutrient dense and provided many times the current RDA levels for most vitamins and minerals. For example, Linus Pauling estimated that the average vitamin C consumption of a hunter-gatherer from fresh berries and other available fruits and vegetables was in the order of 6000 to 12,000 mg of vitamin C intake per day. By comparison, the current RDA for vitamin C is 75 to 90 mg per day for adults.

Rates of obesity and diabetes in some aboriginal communities are up to 50% higher than the North American average (which is already unacceptably high), but experience has shown that reverting to a more traditional diet may help address the problem. For some aboriginals, cutting down on carbohydrates isn't so much a fad diet as it is a modern version of the traditional diet eaten by their ancestors for thousands of years.

Other peoples have had thousands of years and many generations to become accustomed to a diet that is higher in refined carbohydrates. Grains, for instance, were first cultivated in the Tigris/Euphrates region approximately 15,000 years ago. Aboriginals, on the other hand, ate mainly berries, nuts, and animal or fish protein until European trade developed no more than 500 years ago. Fortunately, many native groups are now promoting traditional diets, increased activity levels, and the use of traditional herbs in the prevention and treatment of Type II diabetes in the native community.

Children and Adolescents

According to the NIH's National Diabetes Education Program, diabetes is one of the most common chronic diseases in school-age children. In the United States, about 176,500 people under 20 years of age have diabetes. Currently, about 1 in every 400 to 600 children has Type 1 diabetes. However, because 10% to 15% of children and teens are overweight, increasing numbers of young people are developing Type II diabetes.

In several clinic-based studies, the percentage of children with newly diagnosed diabetes classified as Type II has increased from less than 5% before 1994 to 30% to 50% in subsequent years. By far, most children and adolescents diagnosed with Type II diabetes are overweight or obese and insulin resistant with a family history of Type II diabetes. Of concern is that undiagnosed Type II diabetes in children and adolescents may place these young people at early risk for cardiovascular disease and other diabetic complications. In essence, the increased incidence of Type II diabetes in youth is a direct consequence of the obesity epidemic among young people. This is a significant and growing public health problem.

Type II diabetes in youth has been recognized for some time, but researchers are warning that new cases of diabetes in the second decade of life (teens and pre-teens) are sharply on the rise. This is largely accounted for by minority populations with higher risk and increasing rates of childhood obesity. For example, among Japanese schoolchildren, Type II diabetes has increased more than thirtyfold over the past 20 years, concomitant with changing food patterns and increasing obesity rates. If this trend is not stopped and reversed soon, the full effect of this epidemic will be overwhelming as these children become adults and develop the long-term complications of diabetes.

Herbicide Exposure

Exposure to herbicides during the Vietnam War, particularly Monsanto's defoliant Agent Orange (dioxin), may be associated with the development of diabetes. Agent Orange was used to reduce tree cover to expose the position of North Vietnamese soldiers. Of the 2.6 million people who served in Southeast Asia between 1962 and 1975, 8% to 11% now have diabetes. According to figures published by the American Diabetes Association, this represents as much as a 5% increase beyond the incidence in the general American population. Since diabetes increases with age, the percentage of those affected is likely to continue to rise.

In 1991, the U.S. Congress passed the Agent Orange Act, which established a system for evaluating the effects on its soldiers. About 8500 Vietnam veterans have been financially compensated under this Act, many for diabetes-related health damages. Agent Orange is not only found in the tissues of soldiers from the Vietnam war, but according to an EPA study in 1982, it is also found in the tissues of 76% of the general American public.

(4) | DIABETIC COMPLICATIONS

Diabetics need to be concerned about acute and chronic complications of diabetes. In general, it is the chronic complications that do most of the damage. Acute complications result from some extreme abnormality of blood sugar, causing either severe hyperglycemia or hypoglycemia. The initial symptoms of acute hyperglycemia will involve excess urination (polyuria), excess thirst (polydipsia), fatigue, and blurry vision. Chronic complications result from high glucose levels (hyperglycemia) reacting with different tissues of the body.

Acute Complications

- Diabetic Ketoacidosis   - Hypoglycemia
- Diabetic Non-Ketotic Hyperosmolar Coma

Chronic Complications

- Diabetic Retinopath   - Diabetic Neuropathy
- Diabetic Nephropathy   - Infections
- Cardiovascular Disease   - Gestational Diabetes
- Secondary Diabetes   - Iatrogenic Diabetes

Acute Complications

Hyperglycemia may result in a coma due to the high level of glucagon stimulation, which is a response to low serum insulin levels. Hyperglycemic comas are either diabetic ketoacidosis (DKA) or nonketotic hyperosmolar coma. Hypoglycemic coma results when the patient takes excess insulin relative to what the body needs during eating or exercise.

Diabetic Ketoacidosis

Any disorder that affects the balance between insulin and counter-regulatory hormones can initiate diabetic ketoacidosis. Most patients already have been diagnosed with diabetes before they are diagnosed with DKA. Usually, only older people will have DKA without any prior diagnosis.

Eighty percent of DKA occurs in people with diagnosed diabetes resulting from inadequate insulin or current stress or illness. DKA usually occurs in Type I patients and rarely in Type II patients. Symptoms include rapid respiration, acetone odor on breath, and diffuse abdominal pain. Metabolic acidosis of pH < 7.35, blood sugar levels of more than 250 mg/dl (14 mmol/L), and ketones in urine or blood are diagnostic of DKA.

The most common causes of DKA are infections, myocardial infarctions, and emotional stress. Even localized infections, such as urinary tract infections, including prostatitis, can trigger DKA. Prescription drugs, such as corticosteroids and pentamidine, or hormonal changes can also be triggers.

The deficiency of insulin and the counter regulatory hormones (glucagons, epinephrine, growth hormone, and cortisol) result in gluconeogenesis in the liver and breakdown of fat (lipolysis), which is the basis of fatty acid breakdown that converts into ketones. The high levels of ketones cause metabolic acidosis.

Prognosis

The prognosis for a young healthy diabetic who is adequately managed is excellent. However, when the patient is old or weak and has other current illness (especially infection), or if the acidosis is very severe, there is significant mortality. If patients with DKA have fallen into a coma or hypothermia, prognosis is poor. In the hospital, electrolytes, bun, creatinine, glucose urinalysis, and electrocardiogram should be ordered. Treatment will mainly consist of IV fluids and insulin bolus of 10 to 20 units IV, followed by a continuous infusion of 5 to 10 units per hour.

Diabetic Coma

Diabetic non-ketotic hyperosmolar (NKH) coma usually only occurs in the elderly. Altered mental status is the main reason that these patients are brought to the hospital. The patient's blood sugar is consistently very high and alkaline. However, the most distinguishing feature is extreme dehydration caused by frequent urination. Laboratory diagnostics reveal hyperglycemia equal or above to 600 mg/dl (33 mmol/L), hyperosmolarity >320 mOsm/L, arterial pH equal or over 7.3, and the absence of ketones.

Prognosis

Mortality rates are much more severe in NKH coma than in DKA, ranging from 20% to 80%. Rehydration is of utmost importance

Hypoglycemia

Hypoglycemia in a diabetic is primarily caused by incorrect dosage of insulin or hypoglycemic drugs. It is considered an acceptable complication of drug therapy. However, other factors need to be considered; for example, menstruating women can experience hypoglycemia due to the rapid fall in estrogen and progesterone. Other contributing disorders to hypoglycemia in diabetics include organ failure, hormonal deficiencies, B cell tumor, and hypoglycemia of infancy and childhood.

C-Peptide is the peptide connecting the A and B chains of insulin. It is used to differentially diagnose patients with insulinoma versus factitious hypoglycemia. In hypoglycemic coma induced by an overdose of insulin medication, C-peptides may be lower than normal, while insulin levels are increased. If C-peptide is high, endogenous insulin is produced in high amounts, either from anti-hyperglycemic prescription drugs, such as sulfonylureas, that stimulate the pancreas to produce more insulin or an insulin-secreting tumor. To differentiate between these causes, drug urine tests must be done.

Chronic Complications in Diabetes

AGE Products

The two basic mechanisms of secondary complications of diabetes are non-enzymatic protein glycosylation and the polyol pathway. In non-enzymatic protein glycosylation, high amounts of circulating sugars start to attach to proteins, forming a compound called Amadori. After weeks to years, the Amadori product undergoes an irreversible conversion to form a complex compound called Advanced Glycosylation End (AGE) products.

AGE products are found throughout the body but in high levels in connective tissues, blood vessels, the matrix of the renal glomerulus, and the phospholipid component of low-density lipoproteins (LDL). High levels of AGE are associated with structural alterations within the body, including increased vascular permeability, loss of vascular elasticity, reduced clearance of lipoproteins, and altered enzyme function. This reduced clearance of lipoproteins is one of the main contributing factors to the high cardiovascular mortality found in diabetic patients.

AGE products are atherogenic and one of the main contributors to accelerating atherosclerosis in diabetics. Treating hypertension in long-term uncontrolled diabetics can be a very difficult challenge. It is not uncommon for these patients to be on three antihypertensive drugs and still not have adequate control.

Diabetic Retinopathy

Hyperglycemia will eventually cause the retinal cells to have an accumulation of sorbitol through the polyol pathway, which causes an increase in osmosis. The high levels of sorbitol are not easily able to diffuse out of the cell in which it is produced. This causes a high osmotic swelling, in which water will enter the cell. Due to the buildup of water pressure in the cell, valuable antioxidants, such as glutathione and myoinositol, are pushed out and thereby free radical damage occurs within the eye. This causes diabetic retinopathy.

The progression of diabetic retinopathy may actually begin without any overt symptoms. Eye exam will initially reveal visible lesions. Micro-aneurysms on the terminal capillaries of the retina form quite similarly to balloons. They inflate but burst very easily. The increased fragility and weakness of the capillaries start to leak proteinaceous fluid, thereby causing hard exudates. The leaking of red blood cells form hemorrhages. In itself, this process does not cause visual impairment. New capillaries do not form and the condition is thus coined non-proliferative retinopathy.

This differs from proliferative retinopathy, in that the retinal vessels further deteriorate to the point of ischemia (arterial narrowing and blockage). The resultant ischemia causes new vessels to compensate for the lack of blood flow to the retina. Unfortunately, these vessels are very weak and tend to burst easily, causing hemorrhage into the preretinal areas or vitreous, causing significant vision loss. Diabetic macular edema occurs when fluid from abnormal vessels leaks into the macula. Retinal detachment is a medical emergency and needs to be treated by eye surgeons as soon as possible.

Progression of Diabetic Retinopathy	
Name of condition	Eye Exam
Nonproliferative diabetic retinopathy	Retinal micro-aneurysms
Proliferative diabetic retinopathy	New vessels on the disc
High risk proliferative retinopathy	New vessels with vitreous as hemorrhage
Diabetic macular edema	Hard exudates < 2 disc

Diabetic Neuropathy

Diabetic neuropathy and retinopathy both have something in common: accumulation of sorbitol. Nerve damage (neuropathy) is an easily treatable condition when one understands its pathology. The polyol pathway is also involved in the capillaries of the Schwann cells of the nerves. Neuropathy and vascular disease account for the high incidence of diabetic foot amputations.

The most common type of neuropathy is distal symmetrical polyneuropathy, which involves loss of vibration sense in the toes and loss of ankle reflexes. This can be found on a routine physical exam. Many drugs inhibit the absorption of vitamin B-12 and can cause vitamin deficiency-induced neuropathy that must be differentiated from hyperglycemia-induced neuropathy. Symptoms include numbness and paresthesias that may cause

Progression of Renal Disease in Insulin-Dependent Diabetes

Stage	Onset	Lab	Risk Factors	Treatment
1. Early Hypertrophy and Hyperfunction	Initial diagnosis	Increased glomerular filtration rate	Hyperglycemia Hypertension Stress homocysteine Hypoantioxidants Pharmaceuticals Protein diet Smoking Insulin resistance	*Decrease:* Hyperglycemia Hypertension *Replace:* Kidney toxic pharmaceuticals with natural medicine if possible *Increase:* Antioxidants Herbal kidney support ACE inhibitors
Stage	Onset	Lab	Risk Factors	Treatment
2. Renal Lesions	3 years after diagnosis	Increased glomerular filtration rate	As above	As above
3. Incipient Nephropathy	7-15 years after diagnosis	Glomerular filtration rate beginning to decline. Albumin found in urine more than 0.03 g/daily.	As above	As above
4. Clinical Diabetic Nephropathy	10-30 years after diagnosis	Glomerular filtration rate continues to decrease. Urinary albumin continues to increase.	As above	As above
5. End-stage Renal Disease	20-40 years after diagnosis	Glomerular filtration rate very low. Increased serum creatinine.	As above	As above, dialysis

(Adapted from Selby JV, Fitzsimmons SC, Newman JM, et al. The natural history and epidemiology of diabetic nephropathy: Implications for prevention and control. JAMA 1959;263;1954-59) severe burning and prickling sensations. Pathological examination shows axonal destruction due to the complications of sorbitol buildup.

Mononeuropathies come on with a sudden onset and leave usually spontaneously. They may affect the third, fourth, sixth, and seventh cranial nerve. Truncal neuropathy in the T4 -T12 area also exists. The pain is constant, unrelenting, worse at night, and is often confused with cardiac or gastrointestinal disease.

Diabetic neuropathy, like all illnesses, can cause depression. Diabetic neuropathic cachexia involves neuropathy along with symptoms of anorexia and depression. Autonomic neuropathy, including both sympathetic and parasympathetic nerves, can cause a variety of problems, including resting tachycardia, postural hypotension, bladder dysfunction, and lack of peristalsis in the stomach (gastroparesis).

Diabetic Nephropathy

Diabetic nephropathy is the leading cause of end-stage renal disease. It goes through a very predictable pattern of five stages. Cardiovascular disease and mortality are a great risk for patients suffering from diabetic renal disease. Nephropathy leads to systemic hypertension because of hyperlipidemia and a decreased clearance of atherogenic advanced glycosylation end products.

Infections

Patients with undiagnosed high blood sugar may come into the office for the treatment of an infection. Infections are more likely in diabetic patients due to glycosylation of tissues that causes irritation and increases susceptibility to infection. Diabetics have an abnormal white blood cell defense, in which polymorphonuclear white blood cells have a decreased ability to perform chemotaxis, a reduced ability to degranulate, and a decreased production of free radicals that destroy infections. This makes diabetics more prone to infections, chiefly *Staphylococcus, Streptococcus,* and *Candidiasis.*

Foot Infections and Amputation

Diabetics are especially prone to foot infections. As many as 25% of all diabetics will develop severe foot problems at some point in their lifetime. Half of all amputations in the United States result from diabetes.

Diabetic foot infections are generally more severe and more difficult to treat than infections in non-diabetics. This is due to impaired microvascular circulation, neuropathy, anatomical alterations, and impaired immune capacity in diabetic patients. Most moderate-to-severe soft-tissue diabetic foot infections are polymicrobial (i.e., due to gram-positive, gram-negative, aerobic, and anaerobic pathogens).

Early detection and prompt attention by checking for signs of infection will significantly decrease the risk of serious complications. Although one would think that the vascular insufficiency is the main cause of diabetic foot ulcerations, it is actually the neuropathy. It is speculated that uneven pressure on the plantar side of the foot leads to microtrauma to the tissues, which allows the bacteria to enter and start reproducing. The patient will have no pain due to the neuropathy and thus continues to walk on it, further aggravating the condition. This eventually results in deep soft tissue and/ or bone infections.

Cardiovascular Disease

Cardiovascular disease and mortality are a great risk for patients suffering from diabetic renal disease. Nephropathy leads to systemic hypertension because of hyperlipidemia and a decreased clearance of atherogenic advanced glycosylation end products. In a study of NIDDM in Pima Indians, it was found that diabetics who had albumin in the urine (indicating renal disease) had 3.5 times greater risk for cardiovascular disease and overall mortality than the ones who had no albumin in the urine.

Diabetic patients have a fourfold chance of having both macrovascular and microvascular disease. Smoking, dyslipidemia, insulin resistance, homocysteine levels, emotional stress, and lack of general antioxidants due to the oxidation of LDL and low levels of vitamin E all need to be considered when treating diabetic patients with high cardiovascular risk factor.

The clinical signs of ischemic heart disease in diabetic patients are different than in other patients. This is one reason that thyroid hormone therapy has to be used cautiously with diabetics, due to its potential of increasing cardiac blood flow. Diabetic patients often will have a silent ischemia, making it more difficult to diagnose. Patients may have no pain, just nausea or sweating.

Furthermore, hyperinsulinemia and insulin resistance are independent risk factors for the development of atherosclerosis.

Gestational Diabetes

Gestational diabetes (GDM) is diagnosed in pregnancy and limited to pregnancy. GDM affects 5% to 7% of women during their pregnancies. It is defined as abnormally high blood sugar levels after a meal. The usual diagnosis of GDM is by a 3-hour glucose tolerance test, whereby the mother drinks a 100 g sugar solution. The standard criteria is: Fasting levels < 105 mg/dl (5.8 mmol/L), 1 hour > 190 mg/dl (10.5 mmol/L), 2 hours > 165 mg/dl (9.2 mmol/L), 3 hours > 145 mg/dl (8.0 mmol/L). If a women is higher at any two time points, she is diagnosed with GDM.

Risk factors include a family history of diabetes, body weight above 115% of ideal, and poor dietary patterns. Babies born to mothers with gestational diabetes may be abnormally large, may suffer from jaundice, may have low blood sugar and low calcium, and may experience traumatic births. Women with gestational diabetes are more likely to become diabetic after pregnancy.

Pregnancy is a complex metabolic state. There is a dramatic alteration in hormone levels, including increased levels of cortisol, progesterone, prolactin, estrogen, and human chorionic gonadotropin. The high levels of circulating hormones have been shown to decrease insulin receptor binding. Human chorionic gonadotropin and human placental lactogen also decrease post receptor effects of insulin. Needless to say, there is also an increased demand of fuel from the fetus. This makes it very difficult for the mother to keep up with all the hormonal changes.

From 20 weeks onward into pregnancy, insulin resistance is common. In normal pregnancy, maternal secretion of insulin increases in late second and third trimesters to compensate for insulin resistance. Glucose not only alters during pregnancy, but triglycerides, cholesterol, and free fatty acids are also increased in the blood, as commonly found in insulin resistance.

Risks

The immediate risks of gestational diabetes to the mother include increased hypertension and preeclampsia; the later risk is developing diabetes itself.

The risk to the fetus is fetal macrosomia (increased fetal size).The postulated mechanism for this is due to the high levels of fuels, such as glucose, amino acids, lipids, and insulin. Congenital abnormalities from diabetes before modern interventions were about 33%, but now with drug treatment and insulin only 1.6% to 2% of diabetic pregnant women have children with congenital abnormalities.

Secondary Diabetes

Diabetes can be secondary to liver disease due to the liver's role in producing hepatic insulin sensitizing substrate. Diabetes can also be secondary to other diseases, such as pancreatectomy, hemochromatosis, cystic fibrosis, and chronic pancreatitis. Endocrinopathies, such as acromegaly, pheochromocytoma, Cushing's syndrome, primary aldosteronism, and glucagonoma, are all potential causes of diabetes as well.

Iatrogenic Diabetes

Antihypertensive drugs, thiazide diuretics, glucocorticoids, estrogens, psychoactive medications, and pentamidine all can be causes of impaired glucose tolerance. Virtually all non-controlled diabetic patients end up on antihypertensive drugs due to diabetic induced high blood pressure, and many will be prescribed thiazide diuretics due to congestive heart failure initiated by the hypertension. Unfortunately, thiazide diuretic drugs intensify insulin resistance, thereby further intensifying diabetic illness and creating a vicious cycle.

Associated Disorders

Insulin resistance is associated with various other disorders, including polycystic ovary syndrome (PCOS), liver disease, and atherosclerosis.

Polycystic Ovary Syndrome (PCOS)

Polycystic ovary syndrome (PCOS) is a common condition (4% to 10% of American women of reproductive age), which results in a lack of ovulation in many women. It is also associated with hyperinsulinemia. PCOS can be treated as a condition of insulin resistance.

The term PCOS is used to describe a condition in which the ovaries typically contain a large number of small cysts ("polycystic"). Symptoms of PCOS may include amenorrhea (lack of menstrual period), infertility, insulin resistance, truncal obesity, and hirsutism (masculinization, such as facial hair growth). Hormone imbalances may include pituitary

---

Associated Syndromes and Etiologies

Stress: Stress has been established as an independent risk factor for Type II diabetes. Physiologically, stress causes cortisol levels to rise, which leads to increased blood glucose, hyperinsulinemia, and, over time, truncal obesity.

Adrenal Resistance: Increased cortisol also decreases the conversion of T4 to T3, leading to decreased metabolism, resulting in increased obesity.

Hypothyroidism and Wilson's Temperature Syndrome: These thyroid conditions lead to decreased metabolism that can cause obesity.

---

dysregulation, ovarian, adrenal, insulin excess (syndrome X), androgen excess, and prolactin excess.

Liver Disease

Liver disease can occur as a consequence of diabetes, and, conversely, liver disease can contribute to the development of diabetes. This is because the liver plays a central and crucial role in the regulation of carbohydrate metabolism.

A healthy functioning liver is essential for the maintenance of blood glucose levels. Insulin promotes glycogen synthesis (the storage form of glucose) in the liver and inhibits its breakdown. This allows the liver to store glucose for use when blood sugar levels fall. Insulin also promotes the liver to produce many proteins, cholesterol, and triglycerides. It inhibits hepatic release of stored glucose, stimulates glucose metabolism, and inhibits ketogenesis. The liver is the primary target organ for glucagon, which promotes the release of stored glucose when blood sugar levels fall. Insulin is also broken down in the liver and kidney.

In Type II diabetes, excessive hepatic glucose output actually contributes to the fasting hyperglycemia. Increased breakdown of stored glycogen is the predominant mechanism responsible for this increased glucose output. High levels of glucagon have been shown to augment increased rates of hepatic glucose output. In time, the abnormal glucose levels found in diabetes can result in a number of conditions of the liver, including excess glycogen deposition in the liver, steatosis (fatty liver), nonalcoholic steatohepatitis (NASH), fibrosis and cirrhosis of the liver, gallbladder disease, and gallstones.

Liver Disease Complications

Diabetes mellitus and abnormalities of glucose homeostasis occurring as a complication of liver disease:

- Hepatitis
- Cirrhosis
- Hepatocellular carcinoma
- Fulminant hepatic failure
- Post orthotopic liver transplantation

Liver disease occurring coincidentally with diabetes mellitus and abnormalities of glucose homeostasis:

- Hemochromatosis
- Glycogen storage disease
- Autoimmune biliary disease

Liver disease occurring as a consequence of diabetes mellitus:

- Glycogen deposition
- Steatohepatitis (fatty liver)
- Cirrhosis

Glycogen Deposition

Excess glycogen accumulation in the liver is seen in 80% of diabetic patients. Glycogen synthesis in the liver is impaired in diabetes due to defective activation of glycogen synthase. However, studies attesting to this have been usually performed on animals with recently induced diabetes. In patients with chronic diabetes, glycogen accumulation is seen, and it is postulated that long-standing insulin deficiency may actually facilitate synthase activity. This and enhanced gluconeogenesis may account for the net accumulation of glycogen in diabetes.

The mechanism of cytoplasmic glycogen deposition is uncertain, but is perhaps related to the large variations in glucose concentration and frequent insulin dosing. No correlation between hepatic glycogen content and fasting blood glucose levels has been demonstrated. There is also no demonstrable association between the type of diabetes or the fat content of the hepatocytes and the presence of glycogen.

The mechanism for nuclear glycogen deposition is also unclear, with the stored glycogen resembling muscle glycogen more than hepatocyte cytoplasmic glycogen. Nuclear glycogen deposition was first described by Ehrlich in 1883. It is postulated that glycogen is actually synthesized in the nucleus and has been found in 60% to 75% of diabetic patients. Nuclear glycogen deposition is also seen in sepsis, tuberculosis, some patients with hepatitis (particularly autoimmune chronic hepatitis), Wilson's disease, and cirrhosis.

The finding of glycogen nuclei in a patient with fatty liver is useful confirmatory evidence that the fatty liver is secondary to diabetes, even if the glucose tolerance test is normal. However, other research has shown the combination in obese patients.

Patients showing solely excessive glycogen deposition may exhibit hepatomegaly and liver enzyme abnormalities, and may have abdominal pain and even nausea and vomiting but rarely ascites. All these abnormalities may improve with sustained glucose control.

Steatohepatitis (Fatty Liver)

Hepatic fat accumulation is a well-recognized complication of diabetes with a reported frequency of 40% to 70%. Unfortunately, associated obesity is a frequently occurring confounding variable. Type I diabetes is not associated with fat accumulation if glycemia is well controlled, but Type II diabetes may have a 70% correlation regardless of blood glucose control.

Fat is stored in the form of triglyceride and may be a manifestation of increased fat transport to the liver, enhanced hepatic fat synthesis, and decreased oxidation or removal of fat from the liver. The steatosis may be microvesicular or macrovesicular and may progress to fibrosis and cirrhosis. The degree of glycemic control does not correlate with the presence or absence of fat. The most common clinical presentation is hepatomegaly, and most patients have normal or only mildly abnormal transaminases and normal bilirubin.

CT scan and ultrasound are claimed to be sensitive tests for detecting hepatic fat accumulation. A negative ultrasound, however, does not exclude the presence of microscopic fatty infiltration. A liver biopsy is obviously the best method for detecting hepatic fat accumulation. It is unclear at this time whether a biopsy is always necessary in patients with suspected steatohepatitis. Biopsy probably should be performed when the diagnosis is unclear, although some authors suggest that it is necessary in all cases to confirm the diagnosis and assess the degree of fibrosis.

Excessive fat accumulation is seen in alcoholic liver disease, obesity, prolonged parenteral nutrition, protein malnutrition, jejunoileal bypass, and chronic illnesses complicated by impaired nutrition, such as ulcerative colitis and chronic pancreatitis. It can also occur as a result of hepatotoxins, such as carbon tetrachloride, and can be seen in association with abetalipoproteinemia, Weber-Christian disease, the HIV virus, cholesterol ester storage disease, and Wilson's disease, in addition to diabetes mellitus. A number of drugs, such as amiodarone, perhexiline, glucocorticoids, estrogens, and tamoxifen, may cause macrovesicular steatosis. The amount of fat frequently diminishes with improvement of the underlying condition.

Nonalcoholic steatohepatitis (NASH) is a variant of fatty liver, in which fat in the hepatocytes is accompanied by lobular inflammation and steatonecrosis. The diagnosis can only be made in the absence of alcohol abuse or other causes of liver disease, particularly hepatitis C. In patients with diabetes and steatohepatitis, Mallory bodies, such as those evident in alcoholic liver disease, may be seen. Nonalcoholic steatohepatitis has been associated most commonly with obese women with diabetes, but the disease is certainly not limited to patients with this clinical profile. There is certainly a higher prevalence in Type II diabetic patients on insulin.

The spectrum of clinical disease in fatty liver with steatohepatitis varies from the asymptomatic elevation of liver enzymes to severe liver disease with fibrosis and nodular regeneration. Patients with nonalcoholic steatohepatitis can develop progressive liver disease and complications to the point that they may need liver transplantation.

Nonalcoholic steatohepatitis should be considered as a cause for chronically elevated liver enzymes in asymptomatic diabetic patients, particularly if they are obese and have hyperlipidemia. In Type II diabetic patients with or without obesity, up to 30% have fat with inflammation, 25% have associated fibrosis, and 1% to 8% have cirrhosis.

The morphological pattern of diabetic steatohepatitis resembles that seen in alcoholic hepatitis. However, the histopathological changes in diabetes tend to be periportal (situated in zone I), while those in alcoholic hepatitis are predominantly pericentral (in zone III). It is not clear whether the diabetes is causally related to the steatohepatitis. In an animal model of Type II diabetes, there is a high incidence of perisinusoidal hepatic fibrosis, while in humans perisinusoidal fibrosis often parallels with diabetic microangiopathy.

Gradual weight loss and good control of blood glucose levels is recommended for patients with steatohepatitis because rapid weight loss may actually worsen NASH. Weight loss >10% has been shown to be necessary for normalization of liver enzymes in patients who are significantly overweight. Ursodeoxycholic acid may be beneficial in reducing steatosis and may result in normalization of liver enzymes and improvement in histology without demonstrable impact on fibrosis.

Cirrhosis

There is an increased incidence of cirrhosis in diabetic patients, and, conversely, at least 80% of patients with cirrhosis have glucose intolerance. The reported prevalence of cirrhosis in diabetes varies widely. Diabetes increases the risk of steatohepatitis, which can progress to cirrhosis. Obesity is a significant confounding variable in determining the prevalence of cirrhosis in diabetes. Even with normal glucose tolerance, obesity can cause steatohepatitis and cirrhosis. The lack of a clear definition of diabetes in the past somewhat confounds these statistics.

Biliary Disease, Cholelithiasis, and Cholecystitis

There is a reported increased incidence of cholelithiasis in diabetes mellitus, but obesity and hyperlipidemia may again be confounding variables. Several articles have reported a twofold to threefold increased incidence of gallstones in diabetic patients, whereas others have failed to demonstrate a significant association.

Gallbladder emptying abnormalities found in diabetic patients may predispose patients to cholelithiasis. Secretion of lithogenic bile by the liver in patients with Type II diabetes probably predisposes them to forming gallstones, but this is likely a result of concomitant obesity rather than a result of the diabetes itself. Increased biliary cholesterol saturation has not been demonstrated in insulin-dependent diabetic patients.

There is no indication in the literature that the natural history of gall-stones is different in diabetic and nondiabetic individuals. The relative risk of mortality following acute cholecystitis is not significantly greater in diabetic patients than in the general population, and neither is the risk for serious complications. For that reason, prophylactic cholecystectomy cannot routinely be recommended for asymptomatic gallstones in patients with diabetes. Any increase in mortality may be attributed to underlying renal or vascular disease. Patients with diabetes have comparable survival outcomes from laparoscopic or open cholecystectomy.

The oxidation of hepatic (liver) cell membranes, which occurs in cirrhosis, causes a decrease in liver function. Since the liver is involved in blood sugar maintenance, poor liver function is associated with the development of diabetes.

INSULIN AND DRUG THERAPIES

⑤

Type I diabetes typically involves damage to the insulin secreting cells of the pancreas, which can occur for a many reasons, the most common of which is believed to be attack by the body's own immune system. This damage is typically permanent and irreversible. For this reason, Type I diabetes needs to be controlled with insulin. Nevertheless, management of the insulin regime, with an eye to keeping blood sugars at optimal levels, greatly reduces the tendency to diabetic complications. Even patients with poor blood sugar control and many signs and symptoms of diabetic complications should not despair. Instituting a proper insulin management regime can result in improvements in symptoms and blood parameters for this group of individuals as well.

Type II diabetes is best managed without insulin. Remember, Type II diabetics typically have excess insulin and insulin resistance. Diet, lifestyle, nutritional supplements, and traditional herbs are very good approaches to managing Type II diabetes. If these first-line approaches are not as effective as desired, oral hypoglycemic medications, such as Metformin, may be indicated. Instituting oral hypoglycemic drugs does not mean that you should disregard natural therapies. Many diabetics do very well with a complementary combination of healthy diet, nutritional supplements, healthy lifestyle, and pharmaceutical medications. Naturopaths are well versed in managing patients with these types of programs.

Type I Diabetes

C onventional treatment of Type I IDDM usually focuses on insulin therapy to replace what is no longer being produced by the pancreas. Regular monitoring of both insulin and blood glucose enables the diabetic patient to regulate levels throughout the day, accommodating for food intake and activity levels.

Intensive Insulin Therapy

For intensive care in Type I patients, it is recommended that blood is tested 4 to 8 times daily to assess blood sugar levels before and after eating. The patient is asked to measure the exact amount of carbohydrates ingested or use the diabetic exchange system to make exact estimates on insulin adjustments.

Advances in pharmaceutical treatments, combined with the availability of self-blood monitoring (SMBG) and multiple-dose insulin regimens, have led to significant improvement in giving Type I diabetics better glycemic control. Tighter control of blood glucose levels has been shown to reduce the risk of long-term diabetic complications. The Diabetes Control and Complication Trial (DCCT) showed a 34% to 76% reduction in clinically meaningful retinopathy in Type I diabetic patients who used intensive diabetes monitoring compared to patients who did not.

Nocturnal Hyperglycemia

Although high blood sugar at any time, day or night, increases the risk of secondary complications, this is of particular concern during the night, when most diabetics are not monitoring their blood glucose levels. One way to stabilize levels overnight is to split an insulin dose, taking the first half before dinner and the second before bed. The latter injection will cause insulin levels to peak early in the morning, preventing nocturnal hyperglycemia.

Type II Diabetes

Pharmacological drugs have demonstrated their effectiveness in preventing diabetic complications and in decreasing glycosylated-hemoglobin. However, they remain of limited use in enabling NIDDM patients to achieve tight control of blood sugar levels.

Insulin

Insulin is one type of pharmacological agent used in NIDDM. Eighty percent of the cell membranes in the body become highly permeable to glucose within seconds of insulin binding to its receptors; rapid entry of glucose ensues, which is used in the formation of substrates for metabolism. Thin diabetic patients respond quite well and have decreased microvascular complications.

The disadvantages of using insulin in NIDDM patients include the risk of hypoglycemic episodes that can lead to a coma, and the increased risk of macrovascular complications. The use of insulin can cause weight-gain, which is a problem in perpetuating insulin resistance itself. Because it is usually not effective in obese and overweight patients, only a minority of NIDDM patients can take insulin.

Medications

Sulfonylureas

Sulfonylureas, or sulfa drugs, work by stimulating insulin secretion from the beta cells of the pancreas. Following long-term use, they may also affect extra-pancreatic functions, increasing peripheral sensitivity to insulin and decreasing hepatic glucose production. An advantage to sulfonylureas is the availability of multiple formulations that are relatively inexpensive, but after initial success, sulfonylureas are of limited effectiveness. Furthermore, sulfonylureas are contraindicated in liver, kidney, and thyroid diseases.

The limited effectiveness of sulfonylureas was demonstrated in a study with Glimepiride. Five thousand patients with Type II diabetes demonstrated a decrease of fasting glucose by 43 to 74 mg/dL more than with a placebo. The administration of Glimepiride also decreased HbA1c values by 1.2% to 1.9%. However, after that initial success, sulfonylureas are completely ineffective in 30% of patients. Adequate control in their long-term use occurred in only 20% to 30% of patients.

Primary and secondary failure can occur with all oral agents used in the treatment of NIDDM. One study showed that the rate of deaths due to heart attack was 2.5 times greater in patients who had used sulfonylureas for the treatment of glycemia than in the group treated with diet modifications alone. Currently, there are warning labels for cardiac death on all sulfonylureas and Metformin. However, one UK study found no correlation between increased cardiovascular death and sulfonylurea use.

Metformin

Metformin, a biguanide, is the drug of choice for obese NIDDM patients. A relatively new pharmacological agent, Metformin is believed to potentiate insulin and increase insulin receptor sites, independent of pancreatic function. It also leads to weight-loss, which may be another contributing factor in its mechanism.

The effectiveness of Metformin has been demonstrated in pharmacological studies. In one study, 228 patients had an HbA1c value of 9.43%; after 3 months of treatment, this decreased to 8.7%; after 6 months to 8.3%; and after 9 months to 8.72%. A slight rise in HbA1c value after long-term administration was noted. Although Metformin is often prescribed following secondary failure of sulfonylureas, it is rarely effective.

The most common side effect is diarrhea. Metformin also decreases absorption of vitamin B-12 and folic acid. Patients with diabetic neuropathy may have symptoms associated with both diabetes and a deficiency in vitamin B-12 due to its use. It is important to determine whether the hyperglycemia or the pharmacological agent will present more problems to a patient with diabetic nephropathy.

Metformin is contraindicated in kidney disease and a rare fatal complication of its administration is lactic acidosis.

Alpha-glucosidase Inhibitors

A newly developed pharmacological agent used in the treatment of NIDDM is alpha-glucosidase inhibitors. These work in the small intestine by inhibiting the enzyme glucosidase, thus delaying postprandial glucose absorption.

In a study of 1,027 patients given alpha-glucosidase inhibitors, a significant decrease in blood sugar levels was found. However, gastrointestinal
side effects prevented one-third of the patients from continuing this drug
for 1 year.

In addition to its many side effects, alpha-glucosidase inhibitors are also
very costly, and have marginal clinical relevance.

Cautions, Contraindications, and Side-Effects

When considering oral pharmacological treatment, the risk of side effects
must be assessed since tissue damage may be caused both by hyperglycemia and by pharmacological agents used in diabetic treatment. It is
important to determine which may cause more harm.

Sulfonylureas can cause kidney damage and may also be toxic to the
pancreas. These drugs are contraindicated in patients with liver, thyroid,
or kidney diseases. Interestingly, all three organs are involved in diabetes
(the liver produces receptor sites, the thyroid prevents excessive weight
gain, and the kidneys maintain blood pressure control). In particular,
impaired kidney function in diabetics, resulting from either hyperglycemia
or pharmaceuticals, causes progressive deterioration of blood pressure
control. One UK study that divided subjects into two groups with greater
or lesser control of their blood pressure found that the group with tighter
control had a decrease in almost all microvascular complications: a 25%
decrease in diabetic-related endpoints, a 32% decrease in deaths related to
diabetes, a 44% decrease in strokes, and a 39% decrease in microvascular
endpoints. The tighter control group also enjoyed a significant difference
in the long-term perspective of their lives.

SIADH (syndrome of inappropriate anti-diuretic hormone secretion)
can also occur in the use of sulfonylureas, manifested by water-retention
and hyponatremia. Since many diabetic patients have edema due to
nephropathy, pharmacological agents must be ruled out as the cause of
edema in these patients. In some cases, edema may be relieved by discon-
tinuing the use of sulyfonylureas and using a combination of herbs
(jambul, devil's club, globe artichoke, milk thistle, and nopal).

Despite the use of pharmaceutical drugs for Type II diabetes in the last
30 years, fewer than 25% of NIDDM patients have been able to achieve

normal glycosylated hemoglobin levels. Elevated glycosylated hemoglobin and poor glycemic control are associated with increased mortality. Hypoglycemic deaths due to the use of oral hypoglycemics have also been reported. Other adverse effects of pharmacological treatment include jaundice, decreased RAI-uptake of the thyroid, weight gain, chronic hyperinsulinemia, severe insulin resistance, and possibly beta cell exhaustion. Thus, if the number of diabetes-associated deaths is to be decreased, advances in the effectiveness of treatments are necessary.

LIFESTYLE
COUNSELING THERAPY

(6)

Lifestyle modifications play an important role in both the prevention and management of diabetes. Although it was once believed that diabetes was primarily a genetic disease, it is now known that genetic factors account for as little as 5% to 10% of Type I cases. Dietary and environmental factors play a crucial role in its development. The single strongest predictor of Type II diabetes is being overweight. Even when genes increase susceptibility to diabetes, physical exercise and dietary modifications have proven effective in delaying or preventing the disease entirely.

Knowing that diabetes is largely preventable, altering your lifestyle to include more healthful habits that promote stable blood sugar is critical. If you have already been diagnosed with diabetes, naturopathic medical protocols may prevent complications, reduce or eliminate the need for prescription drugs, and enable you to better control your blood sugar.

This may not be easy. Modifying your lifestyle to meet these requirements can be an enormous undertaking. It may take a lot of commitment and time to achieve your goals, so commend yourself for the work you are doing each step of the way. Even making small incremental changes will offer long-term health benefits.

Clinical Studies: Diabetes Prevention Program

Diabetes Prevention Program Results

In the Diabetes Prevention Program (DPP), a major clinical trial of 3,234 people already suffering with impaired glucose tolerance, weight loss and a more active lifestyle reduced diabetes onset by 58% overall. This is the first study to show that exercise and diet can effectively delay diabetes in a diverse American population (45% were from minority groups that suffer disproportionately from Type II diabetes) of overweight people. In fact, the results were so impressive and clear that, on the advice of the DPP's external data monitoring board, the trial ended a year early so that all participants could have the chance to get benefit from knowing the trial results.

Lifestyle intervention worked as well in men as in women and in all the ethnic groups tested (including African Americans, Hispanic Americans, Asian Americans and Pacific Islanders, and American Indians). Remarkably, it also worked well in people age 60 and older, who have a nearly 20% prevalence of diabetes. Their risk was reduced by 71%. A number of other clinical trials involving lifestyle changes have shown that this type of intervention can delay or prevent Type II diabetes in these high risk group populations.

Pima Indians

Originally based in rural Mexico, the Pima Indians have been extensively studied for their high propensity to develop Type II diabetes. Diabetes was largely unknown to this population prior to their emigration northward into the United States. Their diet relied on hunting and gathering techniques, and they successfully farmed fruits and vegetables. Following their migration, reduced physical activity and a diet high in processed foods caused the number of diabetes cases within their population to explode.

Researchers have hypothesized that this has occurred because their genes are 'thrifty'. This means that the Pima are genetically programmed to maximize their energy storage from available calories.

As their diet changed, becoming much higher in fat, refined carbohydrates, and overall calories, their systems continued to maximize
intake, storing large excesses as fat. This elevated their blood sugar
levels and ultimately led to the development of diabetes. Intervention
programs that altered their diet and lifestyle to reflect their tradition
dramatically improved blood sugar levels. The impact of a North
American diet on the Pima Indians has also been measured directly
against populations remaining in Mexico but sharing similar genes.
This research has offered convincing results that lifestyle factors are
largely responsible for the development of Type II diabetes.

Nurses' Study

Several recent studies have echoed these conclusions. Almost 85,000
nurses were followed by researchers for 16 years. The low-risk group
was identified by such factors as cereal fiber intake, body mass index,
and level of physical activity. By documenting 3,300 new cases of diabetes over the course of the study, being overweight or obese was
identified as the single most important predictor of diabetes, while
lack of exercise, poor diet, and smoking were among factors associated with a significantly increased risk.

International Studies

In Finland, dietary and exercise intervention over the course of 1 year
on NIDDM subjects led to better metabolic control and a reduced need
for oral anti-diabetic drugs. Another study in China of 110,660 subjects focused on preventing diabetes in patients with identified
impaired glucose tolerance. Over a period of 6 years, the researchers
found that diet and lifestyle interventions significantly decreased the
incidence of diabetes, and these results were echoed in a much smaller
study of 52 New Zealand subjects that made similar conclusions.

Lifestyle Factors Contributing to Insulin Resistance and Diabetes

1. Dietary excesses and deficiencies
- High in carbohydrates
- Very high in saturated fats and trans fats
- High in refined sugars and starches
- High in high glycemic foods
- Low in protein
- Very low in essential fatty acids
- Inadequate in fiber
- Inadequate in vegetables
- Deficient in micronutrients (such as chromium)
- Salt intake that is either too low or too high

2. Lack of physical activity

3. Stress

4. Smoking (nicotine consumption)

Weight Management

Being over weight is a major risk factor in NIDDM. As many as 80% to 90% of Type II diabetics are not only overweight, but obese. This is a self-perpetuating problem for diabetics because fat cells secrete hormones that may reduce the effectiveness of blood sugar control. Knowing that weight is a major risk factor, lifestyle modifications need to address methods of weight reduction. These include improved nutrition and increased physical exercise. Reducing stress and stopping smoking are also important aspects of diabetes prevention.

Improving Nutrition

The first step in making dietary changes is to view your diet as a way of life, rather than a short-term restriction. It is important to find a healthful balance in your diet that you can manage to maintain for the rest of your life. One method to help you identify more diabetic-friendly foods is to use the Glycemic Index, a measure of how quickly foods are converted into glucose in your body. By emphasizing foods with lower glycemic index values, you will be able to enjoy a variety of foods while maintaining stable blood sugar levels. A more comprehensive discussion of the Glycemic Index is offered in the next chapter.

Unfortunately, North Americans are bombarded daily with unhealthy food choices, and although governments are working toward more accurate labeling standards to enable consumers to make informed decisions, these changes are slow to occur. The next chapter will help you to develop an eating plan that will allow you to manage your blood sugar levels and prevent diabetic complications, but we recognize that making these changes within our societal context is challenging.

Increasing Physical Exercise

Exercise will help you to lose weight, while offering the added benefit of increasing your sensitivity to insulin. Because muscles are sensitive to insulin, maintaining muscle mass normalizes glucose flow and enables it to be used efficiently as energy. Additionally, exercise is particularly important for diabetics who are already at a significantly increased risk for the development of cardiovascular disease.

Exercise Precautions

Since diabetes is a metabolic disorder, it is important for diabetics to take precautions when exercising. Do not skip meals before exercising to ensure that your blood sugar level is adequate to meet energy needs. You may need to consume a carbohydrate-rich snack prior to activity or pack something to take with you. Physical activity lowers your blood sugar, and if your blood glucose drops too much, hypoglycemia can result.

Be aware of symptoms that may indicate the onset of hypoglycemia, such as shakiness, weakness, confusion, irritability, headache, dizziness, or anxiety. These symptoms, if due to hypoglycemia, typically come on when a meal is delayed or missed, and typically improve when food is consumed. Hypoglycemia may also create a strong craving for sweets or simple carbohydrate, which, of course, should be avoided.

Diabetics are also prone to foot problems, so it is worthwhile to invest in a comfortable pair of properly fitted athletic shoes to avoid injury and blistering. A medical bracelet or necklace that identifies you as a diabetic should always be worn.

Clinical Studies: Diabetes and Exercise

Several studies have demonstrated the importance of regular physical activity in delaying or preventing the onset of diabetes.

Protective Effect

Among them is a study of almost 6,000 male subjects whose physical activity patterns were measured for walking, stair climbing, and sports. The researchers identified a protective effect of exercise in preventing Type II diabetes, especially in those at higher risk.

Exercise vs. Metformin

Another 2.8-year study of 3,234 non-diabetics separated subjects into three groups. The control group was administered a placebo, while the other groups were either given Metformin (a weight loss drug) or assigned to 150 minutes of weekly physical exercise. Significant reductions in the incidence of diabetes occurred in both the drug group (by 31%) and the exercise group (by 58%), with the exercise component clearly the more effective preventive measure.

Consistency

The key appears to be consistency. A study that examined the effect of exercise on insulin resistance syndrome in 79 obese children found that the protective aspects of exercise were not retained once activity ceased. The children were randomly assigned to one of two groups. The first group participated in 40 minutes of exercise 5 days per week for a period of 4 months, followed by an inactive period of 4 months. The second group was inactive for the first 4 months, followed by organized activity 5 days weekly. The researchers found that while regular exercise improved plasma triglyceride and insulin concentrations, these benefits were lost once the children returned to inactivity.

Exercise Routine

It is recommended that diabetics partake in a half hour of exercise every day. Even moderate exercise, such as walking, will offer health benefits, so start slowly and work at a pace that is comfortable. Here are some other ideas to help you get started and to encourage you to continue with your exercise regime:

+ If you are starting an exercise program, it is a good idea to get a physical exam, including an EKG or stress test from your healthcare practitioner.

+ Set your alarm a few minutes early to allow yourself some time to stretch, do yoga postures, or take a quick walk around the block. By starting your day with physical activity, you'll be more energized to continue being active throughout the day.

+ Schedule your activity just as you would schedule any other appointment. You may find it beneficial to find an exercise partner to help you to keep your commitment to be active.

+ Don't forget to warm up before exercise and cool down after. In general, 12 to 15 minutes of warm up is a good idea. During warm up, your heart rate is increasing slowly toward your training heart rate. The cool down is also 12 to 15 minutes, which allows your body to adjust after the exercise period.

+ If you are exercising to lose weight, increase the duration of exercise as your fitness improves, not the intensity. Fat burning is optimized after 20 minutes. Therefore, it is better to do 30 minutes at a slower pace (such as 120 beats/minute heart rate) than 15 minutes at a fast pace (such as 140 beats/minute heart rate). Maintaining your heart rate at or below the training rate helps prevent injuries and overtraining. It also encourages the body to burn fat.

+ Make exercise a family affair. Choose physical activities that everyone can enjoy, such as long hikes, camping trips, or ski vacations.

+ Plan a daily walk or other activity that allows you to talk with your children while you exercise.

- Encourage your children to join sports teams, dance classes, or swimming lessons. Provide supervised park time or a safe backyard play space to encourage outdoor physical activity instead of quiet indoor play.
- Plan family events that are focussed on an activity, such as skiing, canoeing, hiking, or biking. Develop family traditions based on these activities, such as a Sunday walk or a New Years ski day.
- If you can't afford to join an exercise class, rent or purchase an exercise video. There is a wide selection of activities to choose from, including yoga, pilates, power walking, and aerobic dance. Children's videos are also available.
- Make every step count. If you're walking back and forth between offices, put on your walking shoes and do so at a brisk pace. Take the stairs between floors. Do errands on foot whenever possible. Park in a distant parking space instead of circling for a closer one. Little activities throughout the day count toward your daily exercise goal.
- Get a heart rate monitor. This device will let you know if you are pushing your heart and cardiovascular system too hard. In general, training heart rate should be restricted to 180 minus your age for non-competitive athletes.
- Value yourself and your health. Set a positive example for those around you by committing to daily activity.

Stress Management

Stress is an inevitable part of life, but long-term, chronic stress can be debilitating to our health. Chronic stress plays a major role in the development of Type I as well as Type II diabetes. Stress also plays a major role in the development of IDDM complications. A Dutch study of 2,262 subjects between the ages of 50 and 74 years found a positive correlation between stress and the incidence of diabetes. Stressful life events, such as the death of a partner or a move, were linked to Type II diabetes and to increased fat around the abdomen. Researchers were able to isolate the

Strategies for Reducing Stress

Some suggestions to help you reduce stress include:

+ Practice yoga or meditation. Both enable you to focus your energy and clear your mind.
+ Use thermal biofeedback-assisted relaxation training (BART).
+ Keep a journal. This can be a place to vent frustrations and unleash negative energy instead of holding it inside.
+ Delegate whenever possible. This may include delegating work tasks to subordinates or juggling family chores among your children to reduce the number of responsibilities you have. Hire extra help if you need and can afford to do so.
+ Make time to exercise, which reduces stress and elevates endorphins to boost feelings of wellness.
+ Keep lists of things you must do to help you keep track of your accomplishments. Staying organized will enable you to feel more in control of your time and less overwhelmed by the tasks at hand.

increased risk of NIDDM as related specifically to an increased number of stressful life events, and theorized that this is because psychological stress induces the release of stress hormones that boost blood sugar.

Although major stressful life events are difficult to avoid, it is important to manage daily stress effectively so that stress hormones do not continually elevate blood sugar unnecessarily. The secretion of high levels of stress hormones, including cortisol, results in hyperglycemia. These hormones reduce both the amount of insulin released and the efficiency of available insulin. Diabetic control is thus compromised by chronic stress.

Stress reduction was found to stabilize metabolic functions and reestablish efficient use of insulin. All diabetics should focus on reducing daily stress whenever possible, and find effective stress management techniques. Lifestyle counseling and meditative practices, such as yoga, have been shown to reduce stress. Stress reduction, in turn, stabilizes metabolic functions, reestablishing efficient use of insulin, decreasing the requirements for exogenous sources, and making blood sugar control easier to achieve.

In particular, thermal biofeedback-assisted relaxation training (BART) has elicited promising results in an 8-week experimental trial on 40 subjects (of which more than half had IDDM). When compared to the reduction in stress resulting from self-selected relaxation techniques, BART improved the glycemic control of IDDM subjects, decreased diastolic blood pressure, and reduced requirements for exogenous insulin.

Stopping Smoking

Nicotine is known to decrease sensitivity to insulin in Type II diabetics. Cigarette smoke also contains thousands of toxic compounds that exacerbate the free radical damage already accelerated in diabetes. Combining cigarette smoking with diabetes is an especially lethal recipe.

Smoking will result in an acceleration of the process that leads to blindness (retinopathy), chronic foot pain (neuropathy), kidney failure (nephropathy), atherosclerosis, and sudden death from heart attack and stroke. The foremost goal of any diabetic who smokes and wants to regain good health needs to be quitting smoking. For diabetics attempting to quit smoking, it is best to make the transition from smoker to non-smoker as quickly as possible, thus avoiding ongoing exposure to nicotine from other sources.

Strategies for Quitting Smoking

Mark Twain once said, "Quitting smoking is easy. I've done it a thousand times." Maybe you've tried to quit, too. Nicotine is highly addictive – as addictive or more addictive than heroin or cocaine. Over time, the body becomes both physically and psychologically dependent on nicotine. Studies have shown that smokers must overcome both of these addictions to be successful at quitting and staying quit.

Quitting smoking is difficult but achievable – 40 million Americans quit in the 1990s, a remarkable accomplishment. Certainly, not everyone of these people quit for good on their first attempt. In fact, smokers usually need a number of attempts – sometimes as many as 10 – before they are able to quit for good. Don't give up after one attempt if it is not successful. Learning from the experience and trying again has been the path to ultimate success for the majority.

Managing Withdrawal Symptoms

When smokers try to quit, the absence of nicotine in the blood leads to withdrawal symptoms. Withdrawal symptoms are typically both physical and psychological. Physically, the body reacts to the absence of nicotine with dizziness, depression, irritability, sleep disturbances, trouble concentrating, restlessness, headaches, fatigue, and increased appetite. Psychologically, the smoker is faced with giving up a habit, which is often tied to many other common activities, such as talking on the phone, eating, or drinking coffee or alcohol. For many people stressful situations also increase their desire to smoke.

It is critical to be aware of these circumstances and to have a replacement habit at hand. Some examples of replacement habits include drinking a glass of water, chewing gum, lifting weights, or going for a walk. The important thing is to find a mix of replacement strategies that work for you. Some people even choose to avoid the behavior (such as drinking coffee or alcohol) that triggers the desire to smoke, at least for awhile.

Nicotine Replacement Therapy

Most smokers say their only reason for not giving up cigarettes is the withdrawal symptoms. A nicotine substitute can reduce the number and severity of nicotine withdrawal symptoms. Nicotine replacement therapy (NRT) provides nicotine – in the form of gums, patches, sprays, inhalers or lozenges – without the other harmful chemicals in tobacco. It can help relieve some of the physical withdrawal symptoms so that you can concentrate more on the psychological aspects of quitting. The most effective time to start NRT is at the beginning of an attempt to quit.

With no plan or NRT program at all, only 5% succeed in quitting smoking and staying off cigarettes for 1 year. Nicotine replacement increases that to 15% to 25% (depending on the study); certainly not stellar results, but much better than 5%.

Other Strategies

Hypnosis treatments and acupuncture treatments have received positive and negative clinical trials of their effectiveness. Millions of people have used these techniques to quit smoking. In our opinion, you are most likely to succeed with hypnosis and acupuncture by doing a series of treatments on a regular basis during the first 3 months after quitting. It is also a good idea to find therapists in your area who specialize in using these techniques to treat addictions.

Clinical Studies: Smoking and Diabetes

A study undertaken at a medical school in Italy evaluated the effects of cigarette smoking on insulin sensitivity. Forty NIDDM subjects, of whom 28 were chronic smokers, were assessed and researchers concluded that chronic cigarette smoking aggravated insulin resistance. In California, a study of 20 smokers and 20 non-smokers led to the conclusion that smokers are more insulin resistant, hyperinsulinemic, and dyslipidemic than non-smokers. A Swedish study isolated nicotine in cigarette smoke as the major contributor to insulin resistance, concluding that the use of nicotine-containing chewing gum may have the same effects as cigarette smoke.

Family Lifestyle

Children's lifestyles are influenced by parental choices. Your family's lifestyle not only affects your children today but establishes the pattern for their teen and adult years, and their subsequent risk of diabetes as an adult. Some basic changes now can have important and far reaching effects into the future.

For example, an extra soft drink a day gives a child a 60% greater chance of becoming obese. It is estimated that the average teenager is getting 15 to 20 teaspoons of added sugar per day from soft drinks alone. Consumption rates of soft drinks among children have doubled in the last decade.

Children learn by example, so it is just as important that the parents set a good example as opposed to trying to restrict certain foods from the children while continuing to eat them. To be effective, lifestyle changes need to become a family project.

Healthy Lifestyle Choices for Preventing Diabetes in Youth

If you have a child at risk of Type II diabetes, here are some suggestions that can help right away. Ask your naturopathic doctor about the appropriate use of nutritional supplements and herbs for children.

- Drink water or 1/3 juice with 2/3 water as opposed to pure juice, pop, or flavored-crystal beverages.
- Eat whole grains and legumes as opposed to refined 'white' carbohydrates.
- Add chromium-rich foods to the diet, such as brewer's yeast.
- Serve an assortment of non-starchy vegetables in the daily menu, including garlic and onions that help regulate blood sugar.
- Add herbs and spices to the diet, including turmeric, bay leaf, cloves, and cinnamon, which also help regulate blood sugar.
- Eat high-quality protein with each meal, such as fish, free-range chicken or beef, lamb, or eggs.
- For snacks, offer nuts, whole fruits, and protein shakes.
- Eat smaller, more frequent meals.
- Bake with stevia (a natural sweetener available in health food stores) rather than sugar.
- Serve foods high in omega-3 (cold water fish) to help maintain healthy blood sugars.
- Plan family events that involve 30 minutes a day of moderate physical activity.
- Restrict television and computer time.
- Encourage your kids to join local sports teams and spend time outdoors.

DIETARY THERAPY

Diet is the key factor in any program designed for the successful management of many chronic conditions, especially diabetes. Given that diabetes is a metabolic disorder affecting all three food groups (carbohydrates, fats, and proteins), dietary intake is perhaps the most significant factor in its naturopathic treatment. Proper diet will not only play a large role in helping to normalize blood sugar levels, but it will also help provide the proper nutrients to manage the disorder and help prevent long-term complications. People with diabetes work with a faulty regulatory system, and unless they change their diet, a deterioration of tissues will continue, even if their blood sugars remain normal through insulin injections or prescribed medications. Many people with Type II diabetes will, in fact, be able to attain normal blood sugar levels using only the lifestyle and dietary changes recommended in this book.

Diabetes Diet Principles

Diabetics need a dietary program that manages food so as to enhance the body's ability to deal with diabetes and the degenerative problems associated with it. A diet based on eating low glycemic index or low glycemic load foods, with an emphasis on fresh fruits and vegetables and quality protein and fats, offers this possibility by controlling blood sugar levels while nourishing the body. The glycemic index and glycemic load are related numerical systems that evaluate the speed in which a certain food can increase blood sugar. Not only will this diet help people with diabetes attain the best control of their sugar levels, but it will also provide less opportunity for further degeneration. Patients who follow this diet and exercise aerobically for 1 hour a day will be able to have very tight blood sugar control.

A low glycemic diet is healthy for most people, no matter their condition, whether they are in good health and want to remain that way or whether they are dealing with minor problems and want to clear them up. Some people use the general principles of this dietary program for weight loss.

Dietary Goals

Normal Blood Sugar

Because of the individuality of metabolic systems, no general diet can be precise for every individual, but diabetics, both Type I and Type II, should strive for an HbA1c below 6 – or, at least, between 6 and 7. The equivalent goal in terms of glucose self-monitoring would be a fasting glucose (first thing in the morning) below 120 mg/dl (6.7 mmol/L) and 140 mg/dl (7.7 mmol/L) for readings taken 2 hours after eating.

For many, this may involve lowering glycemic index and load in stages until these goals are met. For example, one person may be able to eat foods with a glycemic load of 50 three times per day to achieve good blood sugar control, whereas another may have to limit carbohydrates to achieve only a glycemic load of 30 per meal.

Allergen Free

An individual's diet may also need to be modified based on the results of specific IgE/IgG allergy testing, which is recommended for everyone, especially those people with chronic disease. More and more research has linked inflammatory processes in the body to a wide range of degenerative conditions, including cardiovascular disease, diabetes, cancer, and neurodegenerative conditions, such as Alzheimer's disease and Parkinson's

Food Basics

The nutrients in food are typically divided into two categories, macro-nutrients and micronutrients. Macronutrients comprise carbohydrates, fats, and proteins, while micronutrients include vitamins, minerals, and amino acids.

Carbohydrates: Made up of simple and complex sugars, carbohy-drates are used for short-term energy requirements, providing the largest percentage of calories in the North American diet, usually between 40% and 55% of total daily calories. Carbohydrates include cereals and grains, fruits and vegetables, and, to a lesser extent, milk and dairy products. Carbohydrates, especially simple sugars, have a direct impact on blood sugar levels.

Fats: Made up of fatty acids and glycerol, fats store energy for long-term use, give structure to our cells, and transport throughout the body important fat-soluble micronutrients, such as vitamin A, D, E, and K.

Proteins: Made up of amino acids, proteins are used to build muscles and organs, to make enzymes, and to provide energy in conditions of extreme dieting or starvation.

Micronutrients: Made up of vitamins, minerals, and cofactors, micronu-trients are important for growth and development, metabolism, diges-tion and absorption, and protection against disease. Eating a diet of whole, fresh foods will usually provide healthy people with adequate micronutrients, but processed foods have often been stripped of their micronutrient content, requiring these foods to be 'fortified' with micronu-trients. The diet may need to be supplemented with additional vitamins, minerals, and amino acids to gain and maintain good health.

disease. One simple way to reduce inflammation is to identify and then avoid foods that trigger an inflammatory response. Allergy tests are now readily available from healthcare providers. Dairy products, gluten (found in some grains, such as wheat), eggs, citrus, and soy are common allergens. Avoiding allergenic foods can result in remarkable benefits in terms of energy, immune function, weight management, and blood sugar control.

Positive Attitude

Many people may find this regimen difficult to start and maintain. Don't try to make too many changes too quickly… no more than you can comfortably handle. Look at this program as a goal to strive for. Whatever changes you can make easily, do so. Just increasing the amount and variety of fruits and vegetables you eat is one big step. Another easy step for some may be to eliminate dense carbohydrates. Of course, the more changes you can make at the outset, the better. For some people, making extensive and immediate changes works best for them.

The key is to maintain a persistent attitude. Remember, "Rome was not built in a day" and "The longest journey begins with a single step." What hinders many people is that once they "cheat," they develop a "What's the use" or "I can't do this" attitude. Instead, develop a "If I fall off the horse, I will get back on tomorrow" attitude. Good diet and exercise alone can often work wonders in bringing down blood sugar levels.

Nutrient Excesses and Deficiencies

Strangely enough, the high sugar diet that contributes to the onset of diabetes can also lead to deficiencies of other nutrients. As Sally Fallon and Mary Enig, in their book *Nourishing Traditions,* remark, "In 1821, the average intake of sugar was 10 lbs/year. Today it is 170 lbs, which is one quarter of the caloric intake. Another large portion of total calories comes from white flour and refined vegetable oils. Therefore, less than half our diet must provide all nutrients to a body that is under constant stress from its intake of sugar, white flour, rancid and hydrogenated oils. This, then, can be seen as the root cause of the vast increase in degenerative diseases that plague modern America." This is true for prediabetics and diabetics. Although the total caloric intake in the diet of many North Americans is generally well above adequate levels, the diet is deficient in many nutrients that healthy people need to prevent diabetes and that diabetics need to maintain or improve their current health.

The processed foods many people are used to eating not only have fewer nutrients, they also often require more nutrients just to help our bodies digest them. These processed foods can be a drain on our nutrient levels, acting like scavengers, damaging these nutrients or increasing their excretion from the body. Some experts consider diabetes to be a nutrient deficiency disease because many essential nutrients are deficient in diabetics, including vitamin A, vitamin D, vitamin B-1, B-2, and B-6, folic acid, chromium, magnesium, calcium, zinc, manganese, and the amino acids cysteine, taurine, and arginine.

By eating the proper diet, the dietary excesses that contribute to high glucose levels and insulin resistance can be eliminated. Eating nutrient-dense foods will also help restore nutrient levels and forestall the deterioration of tissues that may continue despite normal blood sugar levels being attained through insulin injection or prescribed drugs.

Free Radicals and Antioxidants

Diabetics need to eat a nutrient-dense diet to minimize or prevent the damage from free radicals caused by their faulty metabolism. Free radicals are highly reactive molecules that create oxidative stress and damage cell membranes, thus promoting disease and accelerating the aging process. They are countered in the body by antioxidants, such as vitamin C, vitamin E, and selenium. Free radical production, which naturally occurs during the process of metabolism, is magnified for anyone dealing with diabetes. Thus, it is crucial for diabetics to receive high levels of antioxidants, both in their foods and in the form of supplements.

Key Terms

Glycemic Index (GI): A ranking of foods based on how they affect our blood glucose levels. This index measures how much your blood glucose increases in the 1 to 2 hours after eating the particular food. The higher the glycemic index numerical value, the higher the blood sugar is raised. The glycemic index can be considered as a measure of the quality of foods, especially carbohydrates, with a lower number being more desirable.

Glycemic Load (GL): Calculated by multiplying the amount of carbohydrate in a serving by that food's glycemic index in decimal form. In other words, glycemic load takes into account not only the quality of the carbohydrate, but also the quantity of carbohydrate in a particular food.

Glycemic Index of Common Foods

Foods that are high in glycemic index tend to increase blood sugar and insulin levels quickly. For a diabetic, foods over 50 on the index should be avoided at all times, except for the occasional cheating. Adding high fiber foods, supplements, or protein tends to modulate the glycemic index of foods, so this is encouraged.

Glycemic index does not necessarily correlate with the amount of carbohydrate levels. For example, orange juice has a higher glycemic index than apple juice, but apple juice has higher carbohydrate levels. Thus, a diabetic should consider glycemic index and carbohydrate levels. Foods that are high in carbohydrates, like flours, grains, tubers, and some fruits, should be limited.

Grain Products

Baguette	95
Wheat bread, no gluten	90
White bread	78
Waffles	76
Donuts, plain	76
Bread stuffing	74
Kaiser rolls	73
Bagel, white	72
Melba toast	70
Tortilla, corn	70
Whole wheat bread	69
Most cakes and pastries	65
Rye flour bread	64
Hamburger bun	61
Cheese pizza	60
Pita bread	57
Pumpernickel bread	50
Oat bran bread	48
Mixed grain bread	48
Cake, banana,with sugar	47
Sponge cake	46

Root Vegetables

Parsnips	97
Potato, baked	85
Potato, instant	83
Potato, french fries	75
Potato, boiled	73
Potato, mashed	70
Rutabaga	72
Beets	64
Sweet potato	54
Yam	51
Carrots	49
Carrot juice	45
Carrots, cooked	39

Fresh Vegetables

Pumpkin	75
Sweet corn	55
Peas, green	48
Peas, dried	22
Green vegetables, all	>30

Legumes

Broad beans	79
Butter beans	54
Lentils, canned	52
Kidney beans,	52
Baked beans, canned	48
Romano beans	46
Pinto beans, canned	45
Garbanzo beans, canned	42

Black-eyed peas	41	**Sugars**	
Pinto beans	39	Maltose	105
Navy beans	38	Maltodextrin	105
Garbanzo beans	33	Glucose	100
Split peas	32	Sucrose	64
Lima beans	32	High fructose corn syrup	62
Butter beans	31	Honey	58
Kidney beans	29	Lactose	46
Lentils	29	Fructose	21
Soybeans	18	Agave nectar	10
		Artificial sweeteners	>5
Breakfast Cereals		Stevia liquid extract	0
Puffed Rice	90		
Rice Chex	89	**Fruits**	
Corn Chex	83	Watermelon	72
Rice Krispies	82	Pineapple	66
Post Flakes	80	Cantaloupe	65
Coco Pops	77	Raisins	64
Total	76	Apricots, canned	64
Cheerios	74	Apricots	57
Puffed Wheat	74	Mangos	56
Golden Grahams	71	Fruit cocktail, canned	55
Cream of Wheat	70	Bananas	54
Shredded Wheat	69	Kiwifruit	53
Sustain 57	68	Orange juice	52
Grape Nuts	67	Grapefruit juice	48
Nutri-Grain	66	Peaches, canned	47
Life	66	Pineapple juice	46
Oatmeal, quick	61	Grapes	46
Kellogg's Just Right	59	Oranges	44
Bran Chex	58	Pears, canned	44
Kellogg's Mini-Wheats	57	Peaches	42
Muesli	56	Apple juice	41
Kellogg's Honey Smack	55	Plums	39
Oat Bran	55	Apples	38
Special K	54	Pears	37
Bran Buds	53	Strawberries	32
Oatmeal, regular	49	Apricots, dried	31
All-Bran	42	Grapefruit	25
Kellogg's Guardian	41	Cherries	22
All Bran Fruit & Oats	39		

Specialty Foods

Tofu frozen dessert	105
Cactus jam	91
Breadfruit	68
Taro	54
Fish fingers	38
Sausages	28
Nopales, prickly pear cactus	7

Cookies and Crackers

Puffed crispbread	81
Morning coffee cookie	79
Rice cakes	77
Vanilla wafers	77
Graham crackers	74
Wheat thins	67
Rye crispbread	65
Shortbread	64
Chocolate chip cookies	64
Oatmeal cookies, without raisins	55

Beverages

Gatorade	95
Soft drinks	68
Diet soda, with caffeine	30
Soy milk	30
Diet soda, with out caffeine	0

Pasta

Rice pasta, brown	92
Gnocchi	67
Macaroni & cheese	64
Spaghetti, durum	55
Instant noodles	47
Linguini	46
Macaroni	45
Spaghetti, white	41
Ravioli, durum, meat fill	39
Spaghetti, whole meal	37
Vermicelli	35
Fettuccini	32
Spaghetti, protein enriched	27

Dairy

Yogurt, sweetened	63
Ice cream	61
Ice cream, low fat	50
Chocolate milk with sugar	34
Skim milk	32
Whole milk	27
Chocolate milk, artificial sweetener	24
Yogurt, artificial sweetener	14

Snack Foods

Dates	103
Pretzels	81
Jelly beans	80
Corn chips	74
Life savers	70
Skittles	69
Mars bar	64
Muesli bars	61
Popcorn	55
Potato chips	55
Most jams and jellies	50
Chocolate bars	49
Twix cookie bars	43
Snickers bar	40
Peanut M&M's	32
Peanuts	15

Low Glycemic Foods

M any diabetics have tried dieting, but the program is often too lenient to help in achieving blood sugar goals. A strict low glycemic diet, such as the Syndrome X diet, developed by Gerald Reaven, excludes any food with a glycemic index greater than 50, and balances good carbohydrates with essential fats and adequate protein. If you want to eat anything with a glycemic index over 50, combine it with low-fat protein, and exercise for 30 minutes that day.

Restrictions and Allowances

The low glycemic diet typically restricts the following foods:
- Simple sugars and carbohydrates (sucrose, fructose, sweets, cookies, candy, ice cream, pastries, honey, fruit juice, soda pop, alcoholic beverages, etc.)
- Refined grains and carbohydrates (white flour products, white pasta, white rice, etc.)
- Most processed grain products (breads, pasta, cornbread, tortillas, crackers, popcorn, etc.)
- Artificial sweeteners (may raise insulin levels)

And allows the following foods:
- Lots and lots of non-starchy vegetables. These should be the main source of carbohydrates in the diet.
- Whole grains (brown rice, wheat, rye, barley and buckwheat) in controlled amounts (total maximum glycemic load of 150 daily)
- Legumes (beans, peas, peanuts, soybeans, soy products, etc.)
- Nuts, seeds, and nut butters
- Fruits but higher glycemic fruits are better if eaten with protein meals or snacks and not alone. Berries are best. No dried fruit or fruit juices.
- Fish and chicken

Recommended Low Glycemic Vegetables		

Highly Recommended Vegetables (Low starch)
Eat as many of these as possible for the best health.

Artichoke	Collard greens	Parsley
Asparagus	Cucumber	Peppers (all kinds)
Avocado	Dandelion greens	Purslane
Beet greens	Endive	Plantain
Bok Choy	Escarole	Radish
Broccoli	Fennel	Seaweed
Brussel sprouts	Garlic	Spinach
Cabbage	Kale	Swiss chard
(green and red)	Kohlrabi	Tomatillos
Cauliflower	Lettuce	Tomatoes
Celery	(avoid iceberg)	Turnip greens
Chicory	Mushrooms	Turnips
Chinese cabbage	Mustard greens	Watercress
Chives	Onions	Zucchini

Vegetables to Use in Moderation (Medium starch)

Beets	Jicima	New potatoes
Carrots	Peas (actually a	Taro
Green beans	legume)	Yams
Eggplant	Squashes	

Vegetables to Avoid (High starch)

Potatoes	Pumpkin	Sweet potatoes
Parsnip	Rutabaga	Corn (actually a grain)

Special Foods for Diabetics

Some foods are better than others for preventing and treating diabetes. These nutrient-dense 'super' foods appear to have healing properties that go beyond aiding in reaching and maintaining normal blood sugar levels. They address the nutrient deficiencies caused by a poor diet. All foods listed here are low GI or low GL or both.

Super Foods

Food	Comments
Apples	Rich in boron, which helps with osteoporosis and reduces the risk of stroke. Rich in pectin, a water-soluble fiber.
Avocados	Rich in monounsaturated fats. Good for diabetes and cholesterol levels.
Beans and legumes	Important for their high fiber content and B vitamins. They should not, however, be counted as a protein. They are a denser carbohydrate and thus should be eaten frequently, but in small amounts – one half cup along with a quality protein.
Blueberries	Full of antioxidants and phytonutrients. Wild blueberries are recommended for their health benefits for diabetics, specifically. In Europe, where they are known as bilberries, they play a large role in the treatment of diabetes. Mulberries also help with glucose management and may be eaten dried.
Bitter melon	Blood glucose lowering compounds. Found in Oriental food markets.
Broccoli	Rich in many nutrients, including chromium, which is a helpful protection for diabetics. Good source of fiber and antioxidants, including quercetin and glutathione. Also anti-cancerous.
Burdock root	Purifies the blood. Use it in soups or juice a small amount in freshly made juices.
Chinese wolfberries (goji berries)	Extremely rich in antioxidants. Especially good for the eyes and kidneys. Can be used like raisins, though they are a little tart. Available at herbal stores. A handful a day is all that is needed.
Cinnamon tea	Aids in lowering blood glucose levels.

Food	Comments
Daikon radish	Alkalizes the body and purifies the blood. It can be used in fresh juices or made into a tea.
Fenugreek	Seeds boiled for 20 minutes and drunk as a tea are good for glucose control.
Garlic	Helps to reduce cholesterol, blood sugar levels, triglycerides, and blood pressure. Enhances the immune system. Should be mashed or chopped into small pieces, allowed to sit for 15 minutes, so oxygen can react with the ingredients in garlic, making it more potent and more easily assimilated.
Ginger	Relaxes the intestinal tract, relieves nausea and vomiting. An excellent source of minerals. Good for the heart and kidneys (helping to protect the kidneys from damage). However, it may aggravate any problems with elevated estrogen in women.
Sauerkraut	Lowers blood pressure, slows heartbeat, promotes calmness and sleep. Positive effect on peristalsis (digestion). Aids in the metabolism of fats. Powerful effect on the parasympathetic nervous system.
Watercress and horseradish	Help heal the pancreas, but should be added to meals in small amounts only.
Yeast and yeast extracts	If used frequently and in small amounts, can have a stimulating effect on the pancreas if there is not enough insulin being produced.

High Fiber Foods

Although food guides recommend 20 to 25 g of fiber in the daily diet, studies show people with diabetes do better with 35 to 40 g. To your diet, add diet nuts, seeds, whole grains, fibrous fruits and vegetables, beans and legumes. If you do decide to add supplemental fiber in your diet, it should be a slow, gradual process to allow your body to adjust. Freshly ground flax seeds are an excellent source of supplemental fiber that provide essential fatty acids and cancer preventing lignans.

Liquid Whey

Liquid whey helps to lower blood glucose levels. It can be used in salad dressings and in making lacto-fermented foods. Liquid whey is made by straining yogurt or kefir through cheesecloth over a bowl in the refrigerator for 12 hours. The liquid left in the bowl is whey. The solid left in the cheesecloth is a good substitute for sour cream, especially if a full fat product was used. Kefir is more easily digested than yogurt because its molecules are smaller. Products made with homogenized milk should be avoided.

Raw Foods

Raw foods, if easily digested, have enzymes and nutrients that are often lost to cooking. High-fiber, raw produce has water absorbing properties that are especially effective in absorbing digestive juices from the gastrointestinal tract. If these foods are well chewed, they can be a good aid in the digestive process.

Raw parsley, raw spinach, and raw broccoli are excellent sources of glutathione, an antioxidant which is lost in cooking. Glutathione helps neutralize rancid fats that contribute largely to clogged arteries. Eat raw parsley or juice it along with other vegetables.

Fresh Vegetable and Fruit Juices

Juices freshly made from vegetables, especially green vegetables, are excellent health promoting drinks, rich in nutrients. If a small amount of a good fat is added to the juice, it will help with the absorption of minerals and will help prevent blood sugar levels from spiking. Coconut oil, coconut milk, or full-fat kefir are good fat choices that also add to the flavor. Be sure to choose some vegetables that will make the drink tasty. A small carrot or piece of fennel will help make it flavorful. You may also choose to add a piece of garlic when making the juice.

Nuts

Rich in protein and minerals, nuts are also a good source of the B vitamins, fiber, and good fat, with strong antimicrobial properties. Macadamia nuts, walnuts, almonds, pecans, and Brazil nuts (selenium rich) are all excellent choices, especially if soaked overnight in slightly salted water and then dried. In macadamia nuts, for example, 80% of the total fat is stable monounsaturated (good) fat, with only 3% of their total as polyunsaturated fat. Omega-6 and omega-3 essential fatty acids are balanced at an ideal ratio of 1:1.

Clinical Studies: Hypocaloric Diet and Diabetes

Weight loss studies with the use of hypocaloric (calorie restricted) diets have demonstrated positive effects on cholesterol profiles. In a study conducted at the University of Australia, some foods, including fish, promoted weight loss while decreasing triglycerides by 38% and boosting HDL by 24%. Research with rodents has found that caloric restriction can also decrease insulinemia.

Foods that Aid Digestion

The best diet goes for naught if the foods eaten are not properly digested and their nutrient content absorbed. Certain foods, prepared properly, assist the digestive process. For diabetics, good digestion of food and absorption of nutrients is especially important because these individuals are typically dealing with a faulty digestive system, usually with some nutrient deficiencies.

Homemade Stock and Broth

Homemade stock and broth made from vegetables and animal bones or fish can contribute to thorough digestion of carbohydrate and protein foods. Because many foods become hydrophobic (not easily mixed with water) when they are cooked, they become harder to digest. However, the gelatin found in homemade meat or fish broth remains hydrophilic even after reheating. Gelatinous broth has been used beneficially in the treatment of many chronic digestive disorders, such as hyperacidity, colitis, and Crohn's disease, as well as diabetes. Properly prepared stock and broth also contains numerous minerals as electrolytes derived from the bone, cartilage, marrow, and vegetables, making them easy to assimilate. Hydrophilic colloids are also present in broth, again promoting good digestion.

Small concentrated amounts of a broth can be eaten at the beginning of a meal or as a reduced sauce on meats or poultry. Animal bones are best if they come from free-range poultry or pasture-fed ruminant animals (cattle, goats, lamb, deer). Most meats readily available to us are from grain-fed animals, which can compromise the health benefits from these foods. Meats from pasture-fed animals are available, but it often takes a good search to find them.

Lacto-Fermented Foods

Lacto-fermentation is a natural process used to preserve foods. Healthy bacteria produce lactic acid, which acts as a preservative that inhibits putrefying bacteria. In earlier times, this is how people preserved foods without freezing or canning.

Fruits and vegetables can be preserved with lacto-fermentation, as, for example, in the production of sauerkraut and kimchi from fermented cabbage. This type of fermentation is also used in the production of yoghurt from milk. Fermentation of dairy products restores many enzymes destroyed in pasteurization, including lactase, which allows many people with lactose intolerance to be able to digest these lacto-fermented dairy products.

Lacto-fermented foods enhance digestion, helping to break down difficult-to-digest proteins and carbohydrates, and increase vitamin levels, a well as providing a natural source of digestive enzymes. In addition, lacto-fermented foods contain antibiotic and anticarcinogenic substances. Lacto-fermented foods normalize the acidity of the stomach. In other words, if there is an insufficient amount of hydrochloric acid (HCl), these foods will stimulate acid production. If acid levels are too high in the stomach, there is an inverse effect. The lactic acid found in these foods helps to break down protein and aids in the assimilation of iron from all foods. Secretions of the pancreas are activated by these same foods, which also aid in the absorption of calcium and provide healthy gut flora.

In uncooked, properly fermented sauerkraut, for example, there are high levels of choline, which helps regulate the passage of nutrients in the body. Sauerkraut also aids the body in the metabolism of fats. With acetylcholine in high levels, there is a powerful effect on the parasympathetic nervous system, a mechanism that lowers blood pressure, slows heartbeat, and promotes calmness and sleep. There is also a powerful effect on the peristalsis of the intestines, thus promoting good bowel movements.

Lacto-fermented foods are typically eaten in small amounts, as condiments, for the most part. If eaten with cooked foods, they enhance these foods by providing a high level of enzymes and enrich the nutrients found in the foods.

Lacto-Fermented Food List

To be most effective in aiding digestion and absorption, these foods should be prepared in the traditional manner, using live cultures, with no preservatives:

+ Sauerkraut (fermented cabbage)
+ Kimchi (Oriental form of sauerkraut)
+ Kefir, yogurt, crème fraiche, cottage cheese, cream cheese, cultured butter made from full fat organic milk (not homogenized milk)
+ Pickles (fermented cucumbers)
+ Beet kvass (traditional Russian lacto-fermented beverage)
+ Salsas, relishes, ketchup, mustards, chutneys, pickled vegetables, marmalades, and other condiments (not commercially prepared with preservatives)
+ Kombucha, lemonade, ginger 'ale' (made with a live culture)
+ Homemade mayonnaise (made with a live culture during its preparation, thus further enhancing its benefits and extending its shelf life)

Problem Foods

Avoid all 'stressor' foods that rob the body of nutrients rather than providing nourishment for it. These include sugars, soda pop, refined grains and flours, pastas, processed fats, hydrogenated fats (trans fatty acids), and all processed foods, including white rice. These foods disturb the physiology of the body, they inhibit the normal essential fatty acid metabolism, they affect liver function, and they alter cholesterol levels.

High Glycemic Sugars
Sucrose
Avoid refined sugars (sucrose) because they increase blood sugars rapidly, decrease immune functioning, increase heart disease, promote dental caries, provide no nutrition, and contribute to hyperactivity in children. In addition, soda pop is high in phosphates, thus depleting calcium and contributing to osteoporosis.

Glucose and Dextrose
Dextrose is a form of glucose. Both are commonly listed on food labels. Glucose has a higher glycemic value than sucrose, and is used as a benchmark value of 100 on glycemic indexes. Both dextrose and glucose should be avoided in order to control blood sugars.

High Fructose Corn Syrup
This high glycemic sweetener is manufactured from corn starch. It is found in a wide variety of commercial products and should be differentiated from fructose, which is a low-glycemic sweetener. There is some controversy as to the safety of consuming large amounts of high fructose corn syrup over time. Many of the negative studies of fructose used high fructose corn syrup, rather than pure fructose. This sweetener cannot be recommended for diabetics.

Lactose
Also known as milk sugar, lactose falls about halfway between sucrose and fructose on the glycemic index. It should be avoided in adults because of the prevalence of lactose intolerance.

Honey
Formed by an enzyme from nectar, honey is a combination of fructose, sucrose, glucose, and maltose. It is not a low-glycemic sweetener. Although honey contains trace amounts of minerals and vitamins, it should be used only sparingly by diabetics.

Fructose
Fructose, also known as fruit sugar, is actually sweeter than table sugar, but the glycemic value of pure fructose is only 20 (compared to 100 for glucose).

Fructose metabolizes at a slow rate, helping to control insulin surges. However, there is some concern that excessive use of fructose (more than 20% of total energy intake) may lead to elevated triglycerides. Recent research indicates that some people may be intolerant to fructose, resulting in diarrhea. This reaction is common after the consumption of large amounts of fruit.

Clinical Studies:
Artificial Sweeteners, Stevia, and Sugar Alcohols

Artificial Sweeteners

As North Americans continue to consume pounds and pounds of sugar, diabetics are constantly searching for alternative sweeteners that won't affect their blood sugar levels. Unfortunately, the most heavily endorsed sweeteners in North America have all been associated with health risks, and many have since been removed from the market. Even aspartame, currently touted as a safe sweetener, has been linked to a variety of side effects, including migraine headaches, memory loss, slurred speech, dizziness, mood disorders, stomach pain, and seizures. Its chemical component is further known to affect brain cell function and may be connected to the development of brain tumors.

To produce sucralose, another artificial sweetener, chlorine molecules are substituted for sucrose hydroxyl groups. Although sugar is used as its base, sucralose is actually a chemically-altered non-caloric sweetener. Because of its chlorine content, this sweetener raises concerns. There are no studies of its safety in long-term consumption by humans.

Stevia

Amid this controversy, a centuries-old natural herb called stevia is emerging as a safe sweetening option. This non-caloric herb is considerably sweeter than sugar - as much as 400 times - but has no effect on blood sugar levels.

Native to Paraguay and Brazil, stevia is now cultivated around the world. It is widely available in health food stores and most supermarkets. A variety of products are now available using stevia as a sweetener, including teas, syrups, toothpastes, and powdered protein supplements. Pure stevia is available in powdered and liquid forms. It is a heat-stable replacement for other sweeteners in recipes. Stevia-specific recipes and cookbooks are available for those individuals interested in exploring its use in cooking and baking.

In North America, stevia is categorized as a dietary supplement, which is the reason that it is not commonly used as a sweetener in drinks and food products. However, there is mounting support for its widespread approval as more and more people become aware of its long history of safe use as a non-caloric sweetener.

Stevia and its derivative, stevioside, are nontoxic. There is no evidence of any adverse effects of stevia use. One study examined the effects of stevia on rats over a 2-year period. When tested for growth, food utilization and consumption, general appearance, and mortality, there was no difference between the group that was given stevia and the control group. Another study examined if there was any carcinogenic effect associated with the use of stevia. For 108 weeks, stevia was added to the diets of rats of both sexes. The researchers concluded that stevioside had no carcinogenic effect on the rats. Additional studies have revealed that stevia has a very low toxicity risk and that it is allergy-free.

Stevia offers a number of additional therapeutic advantages to sugar and artificial sweeteners. Researchers in Denmark supplemented the meals of 12 Type II diabetics with stevioside and concluded that stevioside reduces postprandial blood glucose and may offer enhanced glucose metabolism. An earlier study indicated that insulin secretion could be stimulated by stevioside's effect on beta cells, offering promising potential in the treatment of NIDDM.

One group of researchers examined the mechanism by which stevia regulates blood sugar. Their results indicate that stevioside regulates blood glucose levels by enhancing insulin secretion and insulin utilization. This may be linked to a decreased PEPCK gene expression in the liver by stevioside's action of slowing down gluconeogenesis. More research in this area is warranted.

Sugar Alcohols

Sugar alcohols, also know as polyols, are commonly used as sweeteners and bulking agents in processed foods. They occur naturally in natural plant products, such as fruits and vegetables. Although they share a similar name, sugar alcohols and alcoholic beverages do not have the same chemical structure. Sugar alcohols do not contain any ethanol, which is found in alcoholic beverages.

Some examples of sugar alcohols are the hydrogenated monosaccharides (for example, sorbitol, mannitol, xylitol) and the hydrogenated disaccharides (for example, isomalt, maltitol, lactitol). Sugar alcohols have been designated by the U.S. Food and Drug Administration (FDA) as safe for use as food additives, termed Generally Recognized as Safe (GRAS). Most sugar alcohols are approximately half as sweet as sucrose; however, maltitol and xylitol are similar to sucrose in their sweetness. They are commonly found in food products labeled "sugar-free," including hard candies, cookies, chewing gums, soft drinks, and throat lozenges. Sugar alcohols are also frequently used in non-food items, such as toothpaste and mouthwash.

There are a number of advantages to sugar alcohols for diabetics. As a sugar substitute, they provide fewer calories (about 1/4 to 1/3 fewer calories) than regular sugar, thereby promoting healthy weight management. Their calorie content ranges from 1.5 to 3 calories per gram compared to 4 calories per gram for sucrose or other sugars. Perhaps more importantly, they are converted to glucose slowly, and require little or no insulin to be metabolized. In studies, ingestion of sugar alcohols (50 g) by healthy and diabetic individuals produced lower postprandial glucose responses than ingestion of fructose, sucrose, or glucose. In addition, sugar alcohols are not acted upon by bacteria in the mouth, and therefore won't cause tooth decay. In fact, xylitol has been found to inhibit oral bacteria, and has been shown to prevent tooth decay.

Unfortunately, sugar alcohols are associated with some side effects, the most common being bloating and diarrhea when consumed in excessive amounts. There is evidence that sugar alcohols, much like fructose in fruit and fruit juice, can have a laxative effect. The American Dietetic Association advises that greater than 50 g per day of sorbitol or greater than 20 g per day of mannitol may cause diarrhea.

Over-consumption of sugar alcohols may also contribute to weight gain. This may be the result of a wide misconception (promulgated by many manufacturers) that all sugar-alcohol-containing products are 'sugar-free' foods and therefore free of calories. In reality, many of these products contain significant amounts of carbohydrates.

Some diabetics have also observed that their blood sugars rise if sugar alcohols are eaten in excess amounts.

Sugar Alcohols Analysis

Sugar Alcohol	Glycemic Index	Calories per gram	Approximate sweetness (compared to sucrose at 100%)	Typical food applications
Sorbitol	9	2.6	50% to 70%	Sugar-free candies, chewing gums, frozen desserts, and baked goods.
Xylitol	13	2.4	100%	Chewing gum, gum drops and hard candy, pharmaceuticals and oral health products, such as throat lozenges, cough syups, children's chewable multivitamins, toothpastes and mouth-washes. Used in foods for special dietary purposes.
Maltitol	36	2.1	75%	Hard candies, chewing gum, chocolates, baked goods, and ice cream.
Isomalt	9	2.0	45% to 65%	Candies, toffee, lollipops, fudge, wafers, cough drops, throat lozenges.
Lactitol	6	2.0	30% to 40%	Chocolate, some baked goods (cookies and cakes), hard and soft candy, and frozen dairy desserts.
Mannitol Mannitol Syrup: Regular Intermediate High	0 52 53 48	1.6 3 3 3	50% to 70%	Dusting powder for chewing gum, ingredient in chocolate-flavored coating agents for ice cream and confections.
Erythritol	0	0.2	60% to 80%	Bulk sweetener in low calorie foods.
Hydrogenated Starch Hydrolysates (HSH)	39	3	25% to 50%	Bulk sweetener in low calorie foods, provide sweetness, texture and bulk to a variety of sugarless products.

Sugar Cravings

Sugar cravings are often associated with disease conditions and nutrient deficiencies or imbalances:

+ Candida albicans (chronic fungal infection) in the gastrointestinal tract, vagina, or skin
+ Other chronic infections
+ Eating the wrong fats
+ Grains eaten without prior soaking
+ Eating too few or too many animal foods resulting in an imbalance of protein and carbohydrates
+ Mineral deficiencies
+ Using MSG, aspartame, or too much salt
+ Eating too many high glycemic index foods
+ Stress and adrenal gland problems
+ Imbalanced thyroid function

Clinical Studies: Alcohol and Diabetes

Since diabetics are at a higher risk for heart disease than the general population, it makes sense that they should imbibe in the occasional alcoholic drink, which is known to promote heart health. The American Diabetic Association recommends that well-controlled diabetics follow the same guidelines offered for non-diabetics. This means moderate consumption limited to one drink daily for women or two for men.

One study published in the *Journal of the American Medical Association* found that alcohol not only offers heart protection, but also decreases insulin resistance in Type II diabetes. Although researchers were unable to identify the particular component responsible, this is promising news for diabetics who have been avoiding alcohol since their diagnosis. It is also possible that alcohol has a direct insulin-sensitizing effect on muscle and assists in obesity control.

When choosing the type of alcohol to consume, it is a good policy to choose beverages with high antioxidant content. These include dark beers (such as stouts), red wine, and drink mixes that are low/moderate on the glycemic index and contain a high antioxidant content (such as unsweetened cranberry juice). These high antioxidant choices have the added benefit over other types of alcoholic drinks in helping prevent long-term diabetic complications. If you enjoy chocolate, you might also be interested to know that unsweetened (or minimally sweetened) dark chocolate (at least 70% cocoa) has also been shown to contain high amounts of antioxidant polyphenols similar to red wine and green tea.

Grains

Avoid eating high glycemic index grains, especially if they are processed, not whole, because they may result in rapidly rising blood sugar levels with subsequent high insulin release. Eating grains may also help to create food cravings and resultant mood swings.

Following a meal of high glycemic grains, people with insulin resistance or Type II diabetes will find their blood glucose levels rising quickly, stimulating the pancreas to release insulin in order to lower blood sugar levels. Insulin in the blood sends a message to store this carbohydrate as fat. A chronic problem may ensue, blocking stored fat from being used by the body. Insulin blocks glucagon, which promotes the burning of fat and sugar. Insulin also blocks the production of human growth hormone, important in many important bodily functions, including helping to build muscle and to sleep well.

Higher insulin release or needs as a result of grains in the diet may cause an imbalance in the ratio of omega-6 to omega-3 fatty acids since insulin affects the enzymes that metabolize fatty acids. Mineral balance and vitamin D metabolism are also negatively affected.

Gluten Sensitivity

Approximately 15% of the general population has a gluten sensitivity (gluten is only found in certain grains). It is reasonable to assume that at least this percentage of the population with diabetes has the same sensitivity. Rates of gluten sensitivity have been found to be much higher in people with autoimmune disease, such as autoimmune thyroid problems (Hashimoto's disease). Gluten sensitivity is often diagnosed as irritable bowel syndrome (IBS), fibromyalgia, or chronic fatigue syndrome. People are often addicted to the food they are sensitive to; typically, after complete withdrawal from grains, all physical cravings for them stop.

Detrimental Effects of High Insulin Levels

- → Cause feelings of hunger shortly following a meal
- → Raise blood pressure
- → Raise triglycerides and lower good (HDL) cholesterol
- → Cause weight gain that is difficult to lose by dieting
- → Raise the risk of heart attack and stroke
- → Deplete the body of important nutrients
- → Increase incidence of osteoporosis by causing the blood to be more acidic, thus drawing calcium from the bones in the body's attempt to reduce the acidity of the blood
- → Cause Type II diabetes as the cells of the body become resistant to high insulin levels
- → May be a part of the picture in the development of autoimmune problems and cancer

Condiments

Avoid commercially prepared sauces, condiments, and broth. Bouillon cubes, for example, usually contain MSG or hydrolyzed vegetable protein and related substances, not necessarily listed on the label because they come under the category of natural flavorings or spices. Commercially prepared and bottled salad dressings are full of bad oils, preservatives, stabilizers, artificial colors and flavors, and sweeteners. They also often contain MSG or hydrolyzed vegetable protein or similar substances listed under natural flavorings or spices.

Preserved Foods

Nitrates

Avoid nitrates in cured meats (such as hot dogs and cold cuts) and smoked fish because they are carcinogenic and contribute to birth defects. Nitrates are also formed when high heat is applied to protein and in fresh green juices if allowed to sit. There is a link between increased exposure to nitrates (from agricultural water contamination, from fertilizers, and from preservatives in food) and the prevalence of Type I diabetes. Look for nitrate-free alternatives in health food stores, and be sure to consume only purified nitrate-free water. Nitrates have also been shown to be carcinogenic and to contribute to birth defects. The young are particularly at risk from exposure to these and other harmful chemicals.

Sulfites

Avoid sulfites or sulfur dioxide found in dried fruits, unless marked otherwise, and often sprayed on fresh greens. These sulfur compounds especially affect those with asthma.

Soy Foods

Avoid certain soy foods because they are difficult to digest, unless they are predigested through natural fermentation. The substances in soy foods impeding digestion include phytic acid, which blocks the absorption of minerals; protease inhibitors, which block protein digestion and can create a swelling of the pancreas; and isoflavones, which can block thyroid function and cause hormonal changes. When soy foods are fermented, these problems no longer exist. Traditional fermented soy foods include miso, tempeh, natto, and naturally fermented soy sauce. Soy yoghurt is also available.

Excitotoxins

Avoid excitotoxins, such as aspartame (Nutrasweet and Equal), MSG, and hydrolyzed protein, because of their allergen potential. Some symptoms of sensitivity to excitotoxins include rashes, depression, nausea, ringing in the ears, vertigo, insomnia, loss of motor control, loss or change of taste, memory loss, blurred vision, blindness, and seizures. MSG is often found in fast food, processed foods and packaged foods. Sensitivity symptoms include headaches, flushing, tightness in the chest, nausea, and heart palpitations.

Food Allergies and Sensitivities

Food allergies or sensitivities can be a contributing factor in diabetes, making it more difficult to manage blood sugar levels. Try to identify any food allergies or sensitivities so you can avoid the culprit items. The most common are allergies and sensitivities to dairy, gluten (wheat), corn, soy, and citrus foods.

Elimination Diet

One way to detect particular food sensitivities is to avoid a suspected food for 4 days. Following this, eat a moderate amount of the food on an empty stomach. Nothing else should be eaten with this testing. Take the pulse before and after eating the suspected food. If it rises more than a few beats per minute or if there is any adverse reaction, then eliminate the food from your diet. Some reactions to look for include rashes, fatigue, insomnia, headaches, joint pain, and hoarseness. This test should not be done with any foods that you avoid already due to allergy.

Scientific tests are now available from medical professionals for delayed-sensitivity type allergies to foods. These types of allergies, mediated by IgG immunoglobulins, are 'delayed' in the sense that eating the food may produce a wide range of symptoms up to 4 days after consuming the food. This is a different type of allergy than the IgE (immediate hypersensitivity reaction), which is tested for in a conventional skin prick test at the allergists office. Immediate hypersensitivity reactions occur quickly and can lead to intense reactions, such as anaphylaxis. Delayed type sensitivities are more insidious in their manifestations, but have been shown to contribute to many types of chronic disease.

Clinical Studies:
Sensitivity to Cow's Milk in Diabetes and MS

Researchers at the Hospital for Sick Children linked two autoimmune diseases, diabetes and multiple sclerosis, to cow's milk in a 2001 study. High
levels of consumption of cow's milk may have a role in the development of
both these diseases. In multiple sclerosis, cells of the body's immune
system attack the protective myelin covering of the central nervous
system, causing many and varied neurological symptoms. In Type I diabetes, immune system cells target the pancreas so that it can no longer
produce insulin, leading to the symptoms of diabetes.

In both groups, there was a high degree of similarity in autoimmunity. The autoimmunity was not specific to the organ system affected by
the disease. In the study, T cells from people with diabetes attacked central nervous system myelin proteins. At the same time, T cells from people
with MS attacked proteins in the pancreas. In addition, the researchers
also found signs of abnormal immunity to cows' milk in the people with
MS in the study. Earlier studies reported relationships between these
conditions, such as similar ethnic and geographic distributions and similar genetic risk factors.

Since delayed type sensitivity testing reveals that dairy products are
a very common allergen, testing and possible avoidance makes sense for
all diabetics and MS sufferers.

Good and Bad Fats

After a long obsession with low-fat dieting and avoiding 'bad' fats, North
Americans are hearing more and more these days about the benefits of
'good' fats. These include monounsaturated and polyunsaturated and fats,
and exclude most saturated fats and all human-made trans fats (created
through processing and hydrogenation of otherwise unsaturated fats). The
terms 'omega-3' and 'omega-6' fatty acids are now commonly seen in
newspapers and on all sorts of products, ranging from health supplements
to eggs and even milk.

The types of fats eaten influence the character of cell membranes, thus
allowing or disallowing for the smooth passage of signals through these

membranes. This includes insulin receptors and the passage of insulin, as well as other hormones, such as thyroid hormone and adrenal hormones. The right kinds of fats slow digestion and absorption of carbohydrates, thereby lessening the insulin reaction. Thus the importance of eating correct fats cannot be overemphasized for any healthy diet, but especially for the diabetic diet. It is vital to your health to be aware of the qualities of the fats and oils you consume. Using the right kinds of fats slows carbohydrate digestion and absorption. This lessens the insulin reaction.

Bad Fats

Trans Fatty Acids: These fats increase diabetes risk, as well as the risk of many other serious chronic diseases, including heart disease and cancer. Trans fats become a part of the cell and block the cell's utilization of essential fatty acids, while interfering with insulin receptors.

Trans fats are often found in all fried or deep fried foods, margarines (even soft margarines), commercially prepared snacks, and commercial baked goods, pastries, crackers, cookies, pies, and cakes. These fats should be totally avoided by everyone. They are very dangerous. More than 1 g per day puts anyone at risk for cardiovascular disease; the typical teenager in our society eats 35 g per day.

Genetically Modified Oils: Genetically modified oils, such as canola oil, which is most often produced from genetically modified oil seed, are not recommended.

Essential Fatty Acids

Essential fatty acids (EFAs) are fat soluble acids that must be obtained from the diet because they are, in fact, essential for healthy human metabolism. There are two main categories, known as omega-3 and omega-6. A third type, known as omega-9, is also beneficial but not essential. Omega-3 fatty acids are especially important in the diet because they support the heart, eyes, skin, digestive system, immune system, joints, and brain. They also help fight insulin resistance, lower triglycerides, normalize blood pressure, reduce inflammation, prevent blood clots, and decrease the risk of stroke, dementia, and Alzheimer's disease.

Most EFAs must undergo a conversion process in the body to make them

Best Sources of EFAs	
EFA	*Best Sources*
Omega-3 essential fatty acids	Cod liver oil or fish oil supplements Fresh walnuts (soaked and dried first for best benefit)
Omega-6 essential fatty acids	Nuts, meats, and vegetables as part of the diet, not from added oils
Omega-9 beneficial fatty acids	Extra virgin olive oil. Best used raw, as in salad dressings, so as not to destroy enzymes. Avocados Macadamia nut oil. Macadamia nut oil is higher in monounsaturated fat than olive oil and has a much higher smoke point, so it is a better choice for cooking and sautéing The natural vitamin E levels are also very high in this oil.

available metabolically; however, this conversion process is compromised or nonexistent in diabetics. In their original state, omega-3 and omega-6 fatty acids exist as linolenic and linoleic acid, but require an enzyme called delta 6 desaturase to convert into their useful forms as eicosapentaenoic acid (EPA) and gamma linoleic acid (GLA), respectively. Direct sources of EPA (fish oils and wild game) and GLA (evening primrose, black currant, and borage oils) are thus an essential part of a diabetic's diet.

Omega-6 to Omega-3 Ratio

Diabetics need to be particularly careful about selecting good sources of essential fatty acids and balancing them properly. A healthy ratio of omega-6 to omega-3 EFAs is in the range of 4:1 to 1:1; however, the North American diet typically contains an unhealthy EFA ratio of 20-25:1 omega-6 to omega-3 fatty acids. Diabetics need to eat fats and oils that address this imbalance.

While flaxseed oil is often recommended as a good fat because it contains high amounts of omega-3 EFAs, it is only utilized properly if insulin and blood sugar levels are well managed and nutrient cofactors are present in adequate amounts. Therefore, flax oil is generally *not* the best choice for diabetics as a source of omega-3 fatty acids.

Good quality cod liver oil in the winter and fish oil supplements in the summer are much better choices. Taking cod liver oil in the winter also helps to provide us with vitamin D that we derive from being in the sun. It can be taken in summer as well if you live in an overcast climate or avoid sun exposure and use sunscreen extensively. Be sure to check that fish oil supplements are free of contaminants, such as mercury.

Clinical Studies: Diabetes and EFAs

In addition to the broad spectrum of health benefits associated with EFAs, the importance of direct sources of these fats was demonstrated in a study conducted in London that examined the effects of GLA on diabetic neuropathy. Over a period of 1 year, 111 subjects with mild diabetic neuropathy were given either GLA or a placebo. By measuring 16 different parameters, the researchers concluded that significant beneficial effects were detectable in offering GLA to diabetics with neuropathy.

Additionally, a diet high in monounsaturated fat, such as olive oil, has been shown to increase insulin sensitivity in Type II diabetics. In a 15-day study of 10 subjects, researchers concluded that a diet that emphasized monounsaturated fats and lowered carbohydrate consumption decreased postprandial glucose and plasma insulin, and reduced fasting plasma triglyceride levels.

Key Terms

Saturated Fats: Found in higher amounts in most meats and in regular-fat dairy products, these fats are usually solid at room temperature. Too much saturated fat in the diet is considered unhealthy.

Unsaturated Fats: Found mostly in plant products and fish, unsaturated fats are considered healthier than saturated fats. Unsaturated fat exists as either monounsaturated fat or polyunsaturated fat, depending on which fatty acids are used to build them.

Saturated Fats

These fats are found in meats and meat products from ruminant ani-mals. Studies of these saturated fats at one time placed them in the same 'bad' category as hydrogenated trans fats. If these animals are grain-fed, saturated fat does have a negative impact in raising insulin levels. However, when these animals are pasture-fed, not-grain fed, their fat contains high levels of omega-3 fatty acids and conjugated linoleic acid (CLA), as well as other beneficial substances. These saturated fats are used by the body to stimulate the immune system, protect arteries, metabolize calcium, and stabilize cell walls and intestinal walls. Aim to eat meat from pasture-fed ruminant animals, and be aware that even 'organic' meats may come from grain-fed animals.

Monounsaturated Fats

These omega-9 fats tend to lower LDL, the bad cholesterol, but do not change the levels of HDL, the good cholesterol. Monounsaturated oils contain oleic acid, which provides many health benefits, including protec-tion from heart disease. Oleic acids may also increase the incorporation of omega-3 fatty acids into cell membranes. These oils are rich in enzymes, including the lipases, which are activated in the stomach and facilitate the breakdown of triglycerides into free fatty acids.

Extra virgin olive oil (unfiltered, cloudy, golden yellow) and a quality brand of cold-pressed macadamia nut oil are highly recommended as a monounsaturated fats. Roasted macadamia nuts are an excellent snack food. Avocados also provide many of these same benefits. In November 2004, the FDA began to allow health claims for olive oil, including its heart health benefits. Olive oil also contains many powerful antioxidants.

Polyunsaturated Fats

These largely omega-6 fats are needed only in small amounts. Nuts, seeds, meats (if grain-fed), and vegetables will adequately supply our needs. In fact, if these fats are excessive in our diet, they may increase the free radicals in our bodies. This contributes to increasing our risk of cardiovascular disease, cancer, and premature aging. Excessive omega-6 fatty acids may also have an adverse effect on blood clotting, immune function, and inflammation.

There is no need to add polyunsaturated oils to our diet beyond what is found in nuts, seeds, meats, and vegetables; rather, the key is to add foods or oils containing omega-3 fats to achieve an omega-6 to omega-3 ratio in a healthy range of 4:1 to 1:1.

Over consumption of omega-6 fatty acids, as well as the consumption of trans fatty acids, can interfere with the body's ability to manufacture GLA, EPA, DHA, and AA (arachidonic acid). These fatty acids are critical to many bodily functions, including immunity, inflammation, and blood clotting through their influence on prostaglandin production. To obtain adequate EPA and DHA, include organ meats, egg yolks, fish, and fish oils in your diet. GLA can be found in evening primrose oil, borage oil, and black currant oil and should be taken in supplemental form by diabetics to prevent and treat neuropathies. Butter, tallow, and organ meats are sources of AA.

Medium Chain Fatty Acids

While 90% of the fats consumed in the world are long chain fatty acids, medium chain fatty acids (MCFAs) are more easily digested, so much so that they do not need pancreatic enzymes or bile to be digested. They are already broken down into individual fatty acids by the time they enter the intestines. MCFAs provide a good source of energy and are not stored in the body as body fat, nor do they create arterial plaque. Because MCFAs are so stable and so resistant to oxidation, they greatly help to prevent cholesterol and unsaturated fats from oxidizing.

Extra virgin coconut oil is an excellent source of MCFAs, enhancing the absorption of nutrients and some amino acids, generally making them more bioavailable.

Coconut oil has been found to stimulate metabolism and to help restore the thyroid gland to normal function. This oil can contribute to weight loss and lower the risk of heart disease. Coconut oil is also the best source of lauric acid. Lauric acid is an essential fatty acid that enhances the immune system and is a strong antimicrobial that fights bacteria, viruses, yeasts, parasites, and other pathogens.

In some older studies, coconut received an undeserved bad reputation for increasing the risk of heart disease; however, hydrogenated coconut oil (trans fatty acids) was used in these studies. More recent research using

extra virgin organic coconut oil has found it to be a healthy food, superior
for cooking, baking, and sautéing.

Good Fat Sources

Monounsaturated Fats
+ Olive oil, peanut oil
+ Avocado
+ Peanuts, hazelnuts, cashews, almond
+ Margarine with olive oil base

Polyunsaturated Fats
+ Safflower, sunflower, corn, and soy oil
+ Fish oils and seafood
+ Walnuts, Brazil nuts, seeds
+ Polyunsaturated margarine

Food Selection and Preparation

Selecting the best food and preparing it properly is vital in any program
for preventing and treating diabetes. Here are some practical guidelines.

Shopping for Good Food Guidelines

- When grocery shopping, focus on choices in the perimeter of your
  supermarket where fresh produce, poultry and meats, and limited
  amounts of dairy (such as plain yogurt) tend to be displayed. By filling
  your cart with whole, live, natural foods, you will be able to avoid
  processed temptations in the inner aisles.
- Take your children grocery shopping with you and allow them to
  make healthy choices. The number of obese children is rising rapidly,
  and this is a primary risk factor in diabetes. Encourage your children
  to pack their own lunches filled with nutritious whole foods instead of
  resorting to sugary, high-fat treats at school.
- Stock up on bulk portions of whole grains. Choose brown rice and
  whole grain pastas, flours, and cereals that are high in nutrients and
  fiber but low on the glycemic index. Prepare double batches of

long-cooking grains and keep them in the refrigerator or freezer for last-minute meal options.

- Choose raw ingredients whenever possible. This includes fresh produce, but also extends to dressings and sauces. Cold-pressed oils and vinegar make simple, healthy salad dressings, while sugary stir-fry sauces can be replaced with soy sauce, tamari, and toasted sesame oil.
- Walk to the grocery store whenever you can. You'll enjoy a healthful bout of exercise, and limit yourself to only the necessities you're able to carry home. This will assist you in avoiding impulse purchases.
- Upon returning from a shopping trip, make healthy choices easily accessible. Wash and chop vegetables, and place fruit on the counter to ripen where you'll remember to enjoy it.

Food Preparation Guidelines

Making Stock and Broth

Homemade stock and broth can be made in large quantities and frozen in appropriate sized quantities to be used in sauces, gravies, and soups. They can also be concentrated by boiling down for several hours and then frozen in ice cube trays.

Marinating

In addition to using stock and broth to help digest proteins, another method is to marinate meat and fish in olive oil and lemon juice before cooking. Extra virgin olive oil contains naturally occurring lipase, an enzyme the body uses to digest fats, while the acid in lemon juice helps break down proteins. The meats and fish are thus somewhat predigested, making the nutrients more readily available. The end product is more tender, more flavorful, and more easily digested.

Steaming

Many vegetables are more easily digested and assimilated if they are steamed or lightly cooked. Steaming vegetables neutralizes oxalic acid found in some vegetables (spinach and collards, for example). Lightly cooking cruciferous vegetables, including cabbage, cauliflower, broccoli, and Brussels sprouts, neutralizes the goitrogens in them that can adversely affect the thyroid gland.

However, a diet of primarily cooked foods can lead to enzyme exhaustion and difficulties in digestion. For rich sources of digestive enzymes, look to extra virgin olive oil and other cold pressed unrefined oils, lacto-fermented foods and drinks, freshly juiced greens or lemons, raw egg yolks and dairy products, raw honey, tropical fruits, grapes, figs, avocados, wine and beer.

Making Dressings

Homemade salad dressings are quick and easy to make using foods rich in digestive enzymes. Adding fresh herbs, fresh garlic, anchovies, cultured cream, raw egg yolk, and homemade mayonnaise not only enhances the flavor of the dressing, but also the nutritional value, adding vitamins and antioxidants to your diet. Consider using naturally fermented apple cider vinegar, which is readily available at health food stores. Cultured whey, beet kvass, and fresh lemon juice may be substituted. Using these dressings on a salad helps control blood sugar levels by preventing spikes. There is a 25% improvement in blood glucose levels by lowering the glycemic index or load of the meal that follows.

Soaking

Seeds, grains, and nuts contain substances that keep them from sprouting until the right conditions of heat and moisture exist. These same substances also make them difficult to digest. Soaking these foods overnight in warm, salted, and filtered water solves this problem. This initial preparation should make it easier to digest these foods and to assimilate their nutrients. Apply this preparation principle to all grains, all shelled nuts, and all flours used in baking, as well as pumpkin, sesame, and other seeds. An exception is flaxseeds, if not eaten in large quantity. Nuts may be dried in a slow oven or dehydrator after soaking.

Dried beans and legumes also benefit from overnight soaking. Before cooking these foods, they should be soaked for a longer time than nuts, seeds, and grains, with the soak water thrown out. This process will make these foods easier to digest and less gaseous.

Sprouting

When seeds and grains are soaked and allowed to sprout before they are eaten, their nutritional content is maximized, as well as their digestibility.

This process produces digestive enzymes and releases vitamin C, the B vitamins, and carotenes. Sprouting also neutralizes many harmful substances found in seeds and grains, such as aflatoxins (potent carcinogenics found in all grains); phytic acid (which inhibits our absorption of minerals); and enzyme inhibitors (found in all seeds, grains, and nuts).

However, raw sprouts do contain irritating substances that help to keep animals from eating the young, tender shoots. To nullify these irritants, these sprouts are best lightly steamed or added to soups and casseroles.

Commercially grown alfalfa sprouts have been found to have the salmonella bacterium and may contain a substance that is highly carcinogenic. They may inhibit the immune system and may contribute to inflammatory arthritis or lupus. Alfalfa seeds also contain the amino acid canavanine that is toxic when eaten in quantities. They should be avoided completely. This substance is not found in the mature plants, however.

Fermenting

In the past, lacto-fermented foods were common in traditional diets. However, with industrialization, recipes were changed for commercial production and now vinegar is used as the pickling medium. The product is then either pasteurized or preservatives are added. These changes not only remove the health benefits from lacto-fermentation, but they also create foods full of sugar, white vinegar, and preservatives, which many would argue are quite detrimental to health. In their book *Nourishing Traditions*, Sally Fallon and Mary Enig present a method for fermenting foods that is very easy, virtually full proof, and only requires a 1- or 2-quart mason jar to sit on the counter for 2 or 3 days after mixing the ingredients.

Good Cooking Oils

- Coconut oil or full fat coconut milk (may be used for sautéing and cooking, but not at high temperatures)
- Cultured unsalted butter, made from raw milk from pasture-fed cows
- Ghee made from organic unsalted milk
- Organic unsalted butter

Seven Day Meal Plans

Day	Breakfast	Snack	Lunch
Day 1	Poached egg Blueberry smoothie	Green and red peppers slices with guacamole	Black bean soup Green leafy salad
Day 2	Whole-grain cereal with almond milk Banana	Veggies with salsa	Whole-grain wrap with hummus, feta cheese, green onions, lettuce, cucumber, avocado Apple
Day 3	Smoothie Bran muffin	Olives and pistachio nuts	Tuna salad Orange
Day 4	Oatmeal with low-fat milk, blueberries, and cinnamon	Veggies with salsa	Vegetable soup Salad
Day 5	Free-range eggs Strawberry smoothie	Cashews	Yams Tossed vegetable salad
Day 6	Smoothie Bran muffin	Bean salad	Veggie wrap Orange Juice
Day 7	Smoothie Oatmeal with low-fat milk, flax seeds, and cinnamon	Dandelion greens with tomatoes	Tuna salad Pear
Beverages		Water, herbal tea, diluted unsweetened juice	

Snack	Dinner	Snack
Almonds Apple	Salmon Sauteed spinach, garlic, and onions Oat flour cookies	Macadamia nuts Pear
Sauerkraut with coleslaw	Garlic shrimp Lentil Salad Stir-fried collard greens	Pecans with peaches
Guacamole and veggies	Stir-fried free-range chicken and vegetables Bean salad	Walnuts and apples
Peanuts and raspberries	Eggplant pizza crust with desired toppings	Macadamia nuts
Celery sticks with peanut or almond butter	Poached or broiled salmon Green Beans Salad	Brazil nuts and blueberries
Olive oil, garlic, and mushrooms	Pasture-fed beef or liver Salad Coconut macaroons	Flax seeds and yoghurt
Soy nuts and olives	Spaghetti squash Salad	Celery sticks with peanut or almond butter

Food Behavior Guidelines

- Eat approximately every 3 hours, with three small meals, three small snacks, and a small amount of quality protein upon arising and at bedtime. This will help prevent spikes in blood sugar levels.
- Never force yourself or your children to finish what is on the plate. Eat only until you are satisfied, and wrap leftovers for the next day. Forcing yourself or your children to overeat discourages you from listening to your body's hunger signals and can contribute to weight problems and other eating disorders.
- Never use food as a reward or restrict certain foods as a punishment. This behavior places an inaccurate value on unhealthy foods and casts healthier options in an undesirable light. Choose non-food rewards for yourself and your children, such as a special outing, tickets to an event, or a new article of clothing.
- Children develop their sensibility to taste at an early age, so keep in mind that the typical 'sweet tooth' that many children have can be minimized.
- Find ways to increase the nutrient value of your favorite comfort foods. Mash potatoes with the skins on to increase fiber. Make your own popsicles using a mixture of pure fruit juice and water. Pop your own corn in an air popper. Add ground flaxseed to cereals, smoothies, and yogurt to boost fiber and essential fatty acids.
- Critically review your recipes to see if you can make reasonable alterations that will help you to achieve your diet goals.
- Bake your own muffins and cakes, using whole grain flours and reducing or eliminating sugar. Most recipes work well without a sweetener. This will help you to avoid hidden ingredients in processed varieties.
- Make sure your portion sizes are reasonable. In North America, we've come to value quantity over quality, and our expanding waistlines are evidence of the health effects. A serving of most foods should fit in the palm of your hand. Meat cuts should be about the size of a deck of cards, and a cup of whole grains shouldn't be bigger than a tennis ball.
- Share meal preparation duties, especially if you live in shared dwellings. By preparing one or two meals a week and trading portions (or getting together for shared meals) with neighbors or friends, you'll have healthy and appetizing fare on hand, and save on effort.

- Avoid processed foods, including food processed with trans fats and processed grains, such as white starchy foods (white flour, pasta, white rice), along with foods containing chemicals and preservatives (such as fatty or smoked/cured meats), artificial sweeteners, and refined sugar. Most of the food we eat should be fresh and whole, not processed or enhanced.
- Eat a varied diet to minimize the likelihood of nutrient deficiencies. The more varied the diet, the more varied the nutrients. However, the North American diet often consists of various combinations of essentially the same foods, often wheat, meat, eggs, potatoes, and dairy products. Breakfast might consist of cereal and milk, toast and bacon or sausages, and eggs. A lunch of hamburger on a bun, fries, and a milk shake contains many of the same food choices. Dinner then follows made up of steak and potatoes or pasta. The best diet consists of a wide variety of different colored fruits and vegetables. And the deeper the pigment, the greater the mineral, vitamin, and phytonutrient content.

Daily Meal Guidelines

- Eat a small amount of protein upon arising – for example, a teaspoon of high quality whey protein powder mixed in water, a small piece of quality cheese cooked meat, or nuts and seeds) – and the same just before going to bed.
- Eat a small amount of high-quality protein at every snack and meal. Always add low GI or GL fruits and vegetables. Snacks should consist of small amounts of protein (nuts are excellent protein snacks) with a small amount of vegetables or fruit.
- Eat many servings (up to 10) of low GI or low GL fruits and vegetables.
- Eat only carbohydrates with a low GI or a low GL, except following strenuous exercise or a workout. Then have a higher glycemic index food – for example, a bowl of old-fashioned oatmeal. This is the only time your body can handle the higher GI food without spiking the blood glucose or insulin levels. It is also best if a small amount of protein is eaten with the high carbohydrate food a half hour before exercise.

- Eat only quality proteins. The best are free-range chicken, fresh eggs from free-range hens, and meats and dairy products from pasture-fed ruminant animals (beef, lamb, goat, organic meats, organic cottage cheese, cheese made from raw milk and bacterial enzymes, good quality whey protein powder).
- Eat only high quality fats and oils, such as macadamia nut oil, coconut oil and full fat coconut milk, extra virgin olive oil, high quality butter (organic, raw, and cultured), and organic ghee.
- Totally eliminate sugar and sugar products. Read labels and avoid products with glucose, fructose, dextrose, sucrose, corn syrup, maltose, etc.
- Avoid all junk foods – chips, french fries, donuts, all commercial snack foods and bakery goods. An occasional treat of dark (bittersweet) chocolate is okay.
- Eliminate alcohol, tobacco, coffee, and caffeine.
- Do not drink soda pop at meals or any time during the day. Drink herbal teas, unsweetened vegetable and low-glycemic fruit juices, and water instead.
- Drink at least 8 glasses of quality water.

Sample Meals and Snacks

Recipes

BLUEBERRY SMOOTHIE
1 cup blueberries, fresh or frozen (frozen makes it thicker)
1/2 cup kefir
1/2 cup coconut milk or coconut cream
1/2 tsp cinnamon powder
1/2 teaspoon vanilla
Blend all ingredients in blender for one minute.
Serves 2.

VEGETABLE STIR FRY
2 Tbs MacNut oil
1/2 cup sliced onion
1 clove garlic, finely chopped
1 cup homemade chicken stock
1 cup green beans
1 cup cauliflower florets
1 cup thinly sliced yellow summer squash
2 cup coarsely shredded nappa (Chinese cabbage)
1/2 cup sliced red pepper
2 tsp naturally fermented soy sauce or tamari
2 tsp water
2 tsp arrowroot

·Heat oil in skillet over medium heat. Sauté garlic and onion for 1 minute, until soft. Add stock, beans, and florets. Cover and simmer for 3 minutes. Add squash and cook for 4 minutes. Add cabbage and peppers. Cook uncovered for 2 to 3 minutes, until tender crisp. Mix soy sauce, water, and arrowroot until smooth. Stir into vegetable mixture.
Serves 4.

SPAGHETTI SQUASH SPAGHETTI

1 spaghetti squash, approximately 2 lbs
2 tsp butter
homemade spaghetti sauce
grated Parmesan cheese

Cut squash lengthwise into quarters. Remove seeds, cover with water in saucepan. Simmer on top of stove for approximately 20 minutes, until tender. Using fork, shred and separate the pulp into strands in a serving bowl. Add butter. Add spaghetti sauce and top with Parmesan cheese. Serves 4.

EGGPLANT OR ZUCCHINI PIZZA CRUST OR LASAGNA NOODLES

Slice eggplant lengthwise in 1/2 inch slices. Brush both sides with olive oil, then use as crust for pizza. Bake in 425°F degree oven for 10 to 15 minutes after loading on sauce, toppings, and cheese. Two slices equals one serving. Zucchini or eggplant sliced lengthwise may be substituted for lasagna noodles when making lasagna. Use the slices raw and proceed with your lasagna recipe.

COCONUT MACAROONS

1 1/3 cup shredded, unsweetened coconut
1/2 tsp liquid stevia extract
1 tbs whole grain kamut flour
1/8 tsp sea salt
2 egg whites
3/4 tsp almond extract

Combine first four ingredients in a large bowl. Stir in next two ingredients. Drop heaping tablespoons onto a greased cookie sheet, making 12 cookies. Bake at preheated 325°F degree oven for 20 to 25 minutes, until edges turn brown. Remove from sheet to allow to cool. Serves 12.

OAT FLOUR COOKIES

1/2 cup oat flour
1 cup whey protein isolate
1/4 tsp sea salt
1/2 tsp liquid stevia extract
1/2 cup butter

Combine first four ingredients in large bowl. Cut in butter until mixture resembles fine crumbs. Form the mixture into ball and knead until smooth. Pat or roll dough into an 8 inch-circle on an ungreased cookie sheet. Cut circle into 16 wedges, but leave wedges together in circle. Bake in a preheated oven of 325°F for 25 to 30 minutes, until bottom begins to brown and the center is cooked. Recut into wedges while warm. Cool on sheet for 5 minutes, then remove from sheet and cool on wire rack.
Serves 16.

NUTRIENT THERAPY

8 |

Nutritional supplements are very important for diabetics, for several reasons. Many of our foods are now grown in nutrient depleted soils because of current intensive farming practices. Even organic foods are not as nutrient-rich as they were years ago. In addition, our modern high-sugar diet strips our food of vital nutrients during processing. The digestive system of diabetics is also compromised, making it difficult to absorb nutrients even if they are eaten in adequate amounts.

To compensate, diabetics need to supplement their diets with key micronutrients. The better nourished our bodies, the greater possibility of avoiding the harmful cascading effects from long-term diabetes that show up as cardiovascular disease, heart disease, kidney damage, nerve damage, and other chronic conditions. Taking nutritional supplements may be seen as a form of additional insurance against these devastating diseases.

Highly Recommended Nutraceuticals

Based on the most current research, the following medicinal nutrients, or nutraceuticals, are highly recommended for diabetics. Chromium and vanadium, for example, are crucial in any attempt at controlling blood sugar levels. In these cases, the research is quite extensive. However, these supplements alone will not attain the goals of controlling blood sugar and avoiding further tissue damage and complications without dietary and lifestyle modifications aimed at controlling blood sugar levels.

Chromium

Background

Chromium exists in three forms: metallic chromium or chromium 'o', which has no activity nutritionally; chromium VI, which is used in the chemical and welding industries; and chromium III, which is found in foods and supplements. Chromium III is an essential trace element in human nutrition. It was discovered in 1929 that brewer's yeast (which is high in chromium) increased the blood sugar lowering effects of insulin therapy. Deficiency of chromium has since been linked to a number of disorders, including decreased glucose tolerance and Type II diabetes. In fact, chromium has been found to be a component of a molecule known as GTF (glucose tolerance factor), which promotes insulin sensitivity.

A number of human cases have now been documented in which parenteral nutrition (feeding with a tube) has resulted in low chromium levels, high blood sugar levels, and even diabetic complications. Research has shown that chromium supplementation at 250 ug/day reversed these problems.

Clinical Studies

Blood Sugar and Insulin Control

A number of studies have demonstrated that chromium is effective in treating both types of diabetes. One controlled study of 180 Type II diabetics involved random supplementation of placebo, 200 mcg, or 1000 mcg of chromium as picolinate every day or a period of 4 months. Fasting and 2-hour glucose levels (after glucose challenge) were measured. At 2 months and 4 months, these levels decreased significantly in the 1000 mcg group, while the 200 mcg group had no significant drop. As well, after 4 months, nearly all of the diabetes patients in the higher dose group no longer had traditional signs and symptoms of diabetes. Their blood sugar and insulin levels dropped to near normal – something that pharmaceutical medications rarely achieve. The 1000 mcg dosage also led to a significant decrease in average blood sugar levels to normal or near normal levels (as measured by the gold standard test known as HbA1c) and cholesterol levels after the 2 months of treatment, which was not seen in the group receiving the lower dose.

In another study, 162 diabetics (48 Type-I diabetes, 114 Type-II) were given 200 mcg/day of chromium picolinate daily. Seventy-one percent of the Type I patients responded positively, allowing an overall 30% decrease of their insulin dose. This study shows that even those diabetics who inject insulin and/or are in the later stages of diabetes respond positively to chromium supplementation. Many diabetics have trouble with good blood sugar control; in this study, blood sugar control also responded positively, improving as soon as quickly as 10 days after the beginning of treatment.

The chronic use of corticosteroids can result in high blood sugar levels and insulin imbalances. Chromium supplementation was investigated in patients with diabetes caused by the therapeutic use of these medications. At a dose of 600 mcg per day, chromium picolinate was effective in lowering blood glucose from an average of 13.9 mM/L to 8.3 mM/L in 47 of 50 patients. Patients were also able to reduce insulin and/or hypoglycemic medications by half within 1 week of beginning chromium supplementation.

Gestational Diabetes
Gestational diabetes is the most common problem complicating pregnancy today, affecting an estimated 135,000 women. This condition poses a risk to both the mother and the infant, as high levels of blood sugar in the pregnant woman cross the placenta, triggering the beginnings of insulin resistance in the womb. The child is then predisposed to be overweight and develop insulin resistance later in life. If the child is female, she is more likely to develop gestational diabetes during her own pregnancy. Pregnancy is a state of chromium wasting, so it seems logical that intake should be increased during pregnancy. Most prenatal vitamins, unfortunately, contain no or little chromium.

In a trial of 20 women with gestational diabetes mellitus, the effect of chromium supplementation was investigated. The women were given either 4 mcg/kg body weight or 8 mcg/kg body weight of chromium picolinate supplement or placebo. At baseline, the three groups did not differ for insulin, C-peptide, or glucose levels at the fasting and 1-hour time point after the 100 g oral glucose challenge test. After 8 weeks, those who were given chromium supplements had significantly lower fasting glucose and insulin levels compared with their own baseline levels and with the placebo group. The 8 mcg/kg/day group had significantly lower postprandial (after meal) glucose levels than the 4 mcg/kg group. The authors concluded that chromium supplementation for gestational diabetic women improves glucose and lowers hypoinsulinemia.

It has been postulated that nutritional chromium levels may be depleted in women who develop GDM. In one study, hair chromium concentrations were measured in normal and diabetic pregnant women by atomic-absorption spectroscopy. Fifty-two women had a second hair sample taken later during pregnancy that showed a significant decrease in hair chromium levels. However, this decrease was confirmed only for the diabetic pregnant group. It was suggested that impaired utilization of chromium may be a possible cause of gestational diabetes mellitus.

The utility of chromium therapy in the treatment of gestation diabetes has also been studied. A dose of 8 mcg/kg/day (or 600 ug/day for a 75 kg woman), 4 mcg/kg/day, or placebo was given to gestational diabetic women. At baseline, the three groups did not differ for insulin, C-peptide, or glucose levels at the fasting and 1-hour time point after the 100 g oral glucose challenge test. After 8 weeks, the two chromium-supplemented groups had significantly lower glucose and insulin levels compared to their baseline levels and to those of the placebo group. The 8 mcg chromium group had significantly lower postprandial glucose levels than the 4 mcg chromium group. The authors concluded that chromium supplementation for gestational diabetic women improves glucose intolerance and lowers hyperinsulinemia.

Dosage

Chromium helps insulin work more efficiently to allow blood glucose to move from the blood into the cells. The Recommended Daily Allowance (RDA) for chromium is 50 to 200 mcg of chromium per day. This may be reasonable for the average healthy person with no personal or family history of diabetes, but higher amounts are likely needed for people with conditions involving insulin resistance and control problems, such as Type II diabetes or Type I diabetes.

Type II diabetes patients who have taken 200 mcg per day of chromium have had some improvement in their condition in the longer term, but not the faster and more pronounced results in those who have taken 1000 mcg per day. Add to this is the fact that the majority of North Americans do not get the minimum Recommended Dietary Intake (RDI) of chromium from their diets and it becomes apparent that lack of chromium may be contributing to the epidemic of diabetes. The amount of chromium people need varies depending on the types of food eaten and their state of health. Patients with Type II diabetes and insulin resistance/syndrome X have greater excretion of chromium, lower tissue levels of chromium, and less of an ability to utilize it in the body.

The U.S. Environmental Protection Agency (EPA) has calculated an RfD for chromium (III) at 70 mg per day (note this is "mg," 1000X more than "mcg"). The RfD is "an estimate of a daily oral exposure to the human population (including sensitive subgroups) that is likely to be without an appreciable risk of deleterious effects during a lifetime." This RfD reflects a staggering 350 times the RDI of 50 to 200 mcg. The ratio of RfD to ESADDI is less than 2 for zinc, about 2 for manganese, and about 6 for selenium, as compared to 350 for chromium. This suggests dietary supplementation of chromium may be greatly underdosed. Based on the fact that short-term chromium supplementation of 1000 mcg per day was found safe and effective in a number of scientific studies, this seems like a reasonable starting dose for diabetics and those with insulin resistance. Chromium therapy should only be undertaken with the guidance of a healthcare practitioner familiar with its use.

Safety and Side Effects

Toxicity of chromium has been almost exclusively linked to the chromium VI (hexavalent) form. Nutritional chromium (III) is found naturally in many foods, including meats, fish, whole grains, nuts, seeds, romaine lettuce, tomatoes, onions, and brewer's yeast. Nutritional supplements are available in various complexed forms, such as picolinate, polynicotinate, and citrate. The use of 1000 mcg/day chromium as picolinate in 180 Type II diabetic patients for a period of 4 months showed no toxic reactions in any of the patients. Furthermore, no toxicity has been reported clinically in doses up to 5000 mcg per day of chromium nicotinate.

Vanadium

Background

Vanadium, named after Vanadis, the Norse goddess of beauty, is a trace mineral associated with blood sugar regulation. In fact, prior to the discovery of insulin in 1922, vanadium was used for the control of blood sugar. Vanadium is believed to regulate fasting blood sugar levels and improve receptor sensitivity to insulin. Some evidence suggests that vanadium supports vital metabolic processes because of its ability to mimic the actions of insulin. In addition, in animal models, vanadium appears to decrease appetite and body weight in insulin-resistant animals.

Clinical Studies

Insulin Sensitivity

A number of small human studies have confirmed the effectiveness of vanadium in improving insulin sensitivity. In one small single-blind, placebo-controlled study of the effect of vanadyl sulfate on eight subjects with Type II diabetes, treated subjects received 50 mg vanadyl sulfate twice daily for 4 weeks. This was followed by a 4-week wash out placebo phase. Improvements in fasting glucose and hepatic insulin resistance followed the treatment period and were sustained throughout the placebo period.

In another trial, 100 mg vanadyl sulfate was given daily for 3 weeks to moderately obese Type II diabetic and non-diabetic subjects. A decrease in fasting plasma glucose was observed, as well as a significant improvement in insulin sensitivity in the diabetic subjects. The authors concluded that at this dose vanadyl sulfate was capable of improving insulin sensitivity in Type II diabetic subjects. However, no change was noted in insulin sensitivity among obese, non-diabetics.

In another trial of vanadium, 11 Type II diabetic patients were treated with vanadium sulfate at a higher dose (150 mg per day) and for a longer period of time (6 weeks) than in previous studies. Before and after treatment, insulin secretion was tested during an oral glucose tolerance test. Treatment with vanadium significantly improved glycemic control. Fasting plasma glucose (FPG) decreased from an average of 194 to 155 mg/dL, hemoglobin A1c decreased from an average of 8.1 to 7.6, and average fructosamine decreased from 348 to 293. Vanadyl sulfate treatment also lowered the plasma total cholesterol from 223 to 202 on average. The authors concluded that vanadium sulfate for 6 weeks improves insulin sensitivity in Type II diabetics.

Dosage

Absorption of dietary vanadium and supplemental vanadium is poor. It is estimated that less than 5% of dietary vanadium is absorbed. Organic forms of vanadium, such as bis-glycinato oxovanadium (BGOV), are recognized as being more absorbable, in the range of approximately 50%. BGOV is an organically bound, bioavailable form of vanadium complexed with the amino acid glycine. Organic forms of supplemental vanadium have been shown to reduce the chances of gastrointestinal side effects seen with vanadium sulfate supplementation.

The daily dietary intake in humans has been estimated to vary from 10 mcg to 2 mg of elemental vanadium, depending on the environmental sources of this mineral in the air, water, and food of the particular region tested. In animals, vanadium has been shown essential (1 to 10 mcg vanadium per gram of diet). Organic forms of vanadium, as opposed to the inorganic sulfate salt of vanadium, are recognized as safer, more absorbable, and better able to deliver a therapeutic effect.

More research on vanadium is needed to establish an accurate dose/response for the treatment of insulin resistance. Based on current evidence, doses of vanadium from organic sources in the range of 1 to 10 mg per day short term (up to 1 month) and 0.5-2 mg per day long term seem reasonable. Vanadium therapy should only be undertaken with the guidance of a healthcare practitioner familiar with its use.

Safety and Side Effects

Based on available research, vanadyl sulfate appears to be a useful and safe intervention for Type II diabetic individuals with insulin resistance. In humans, administration of vanadium to athletes for up to 12 weeks at a dose of 225 mcg per pound of body weight (33.75 g per day for a 150-lb person) did not result in any toxicity. Further studies evaluating the long-term safety of vanadium compounds in humans is recommended.

Alpha-lipoic Acid

Background

Alpha-lipoic acid is sulfur-containing free radical scavenger found in the cells of humans and in a variety of foods, such as spinach, broccoli, yeast, liver, kidney, and heart. It has been called a 'universal' antioxidant because it is both fat- and water-soluble. Not only is lipoic acid an antioxidant on its own, but it has also been shown to recycle other antioxidants, such as vitamins E and C. It can also chelate with toxic metals, such as mercury, and remove them from the body.

Lipoic acid is approved in Germany for clinical use in the management of diabetic neuropathy. Alpha-lipoic acid has also been used to reduce cell damage associated with mushroom poisoning, radiation, and alcoholic hepatitis. Depletion of lipoic acid has been documented in diabetics, patients with heart disease, and people with liver cirrhosis.

Clinical Studies

Research on lipoic acid supplementation has shown improvements in glucose metabolism, reduced glycosylation of proteins (such as HbA1c), improved blood flow to peripheral nerves, and stimulation of nerve cell regeneration.

Diabetic Neuropathy

Diabetic neuropathy represents a major health problem. A growing body of evidence suggests that oxidative stress resulting from enhanced free-radical formation is one of the causes of diabetic neuropathy. Seven controlled randomized clinical trials of thioctic acid in patients with diabetic neuropathy have been using different study designs, durations of treatment, doses, sample sizes, and patient populations. A comprehensive analysis of these trials confirmed the favorable effects of thioctic acid based on the highest level of evidence (Class Ia). The following conclusions were drawn from this analysis. Short-term treatment for 3 weeks using intravenous lipoic acid 600 mg per day reduces the chief symptoms of diabetic polyneuropathy. This effect on neuropathic symptoms is accompanied by an improvement of neuropathic deficits, suggesting potential for the drug to influence underlying neuropathy favorably. Oral treatment for 4 to 7 months tends to reduce neuropathic deficits and improve cardiac autonomic neuropathy.

Clinical and post-marketing surveillance studies have revealed a highly favorable safety profile of lipoic acid.

Another systematic review done in Germany of 15 trials concluded that short-term treatment with alpha-lipoic acid, 600 mg per day, reduced the symptoms of diabetic neuropathy. These conclusions were mainly based on the results of four randomized, double-blind, placebo-controlled studies entitled ALADIN (Alpha Lipoic Acid in Diabetic Neuropathy). In the first ALADIN study, 328 patients with Type II diabetes mellitus and symptomatic peripheral neuropathy were randomly assigned to 100, 600, or 1,200 mg per day of parenteral (IV) alpha-lipoic acid or placebo. After 3 weeks, the patients who completed the study and had received the 600 and 1200 mg/d doses of alpha-lipoic acid had statistically significant improvements in pain, tingling, and numbness compared with placebo.

In the follow-up ALADIN II study, oral alpha-lipoic acid, 600 or 1200 mg per day, was given to 65 patients with Type II and Type II diabetes and symptomatic neuropathy. After 2 years, both doses of alpha-lipoic acid showed an increase in nerve conduction velocity compared with placebo. However, severity of symptoms was not improved, based on a series of physical tests.

ALADIN III examined the effects of short-term treatment with parenteral (IV) alpha-lipoic acid, followed by extended treatment with oral alpha-lipoic acid. In this trial, 503 patients with Type II diabetes and symptomatic peripheral neuropathy were placed in one of three treatment groups: (1) 600 mg per day parenteral alpha-lipoic acid for 3 weeks, then 1800 mg per day of oral alpha-lipoic acid for 6 months; (2) 600 mg per day parenteral alpha-lipoic acid for 3 weeks, then an indistinguishable oral placebo for 6 months; or (3) parenteral placebo for 3 weeks, then oral placebo for 3 months. Neuropathic deficits were significantly reduced in patients receiving parenteral alpha-lipoic acid at 3 weeks. After 6 months of treatment with oral alpha-lipoic acid, a decrease in neuropathy impairment scores was observed.

Finally, the ORPIL study found that oral administration of 1800 mg per day of alpha-lipoic acid reduced neuropathic deficits and symptoms in 22 patients with Type II diabetes and symptomatic polyneuropathy during a 3-week period.

Insulin Resistance

Experimental trials have also provided evidence that lipoic acid might be useful in the treatment of insulin resistance in humans. For example, a 4-week placebo controlled multicenter pilot study was done to determine the effectiveness of oral treatment with lipoic acid on insulin sensitivity in people with Type II diabetes. Seventy-four patients were randomized either to placebo or to treatment consisting of lipoic acid in doses of either 600 mg once daily, twice daily, or three times daily. Prior to treatment, all four groups had comparable degrees of hyperglycemia and insulin sensitivity. Although not every treated subject experienced improvements, a mean increase of 27% in insulin-stimulated glucose disposal was observed among subjects receiving lipoic acid supplementation. In other words, treatment with lipoic acid improved the efficiency with which insulin worked in these patients in only 4 weeks.

Dosage

In clinical trials, significant improvements in nerve conduction velocity with oral doses of 600 to 1200 mg per day for 2 years have been observed. Symptom improvement was also observed using 1800 mg per day orally for 3 weeks. The optimal dose for oral dosing is currently unknown, but a reasonable approach may be a loading dose of 1800mg per day for 3 weeks, followed by a maintenance dose of 600 to 1200 mg per day. Of course, reduction of total body free radical load with other antioxidant nutrients and better glucose control should theoretically work synergistically with lipoic acid supplementation to improve symptoms. The interventions mentioned above using lipoic acid involved no other additional interventions. Alpha-lipoic acid therapy should only be undertaken with the guidance of a healthcare practitioner familiar with its use.

Safety and Side Effects

Clinical studies to date have indicated that alpha-lipoic acid has a favorable safety and side effect profile. Adverse effects tend to be mild and include headache, skin rash, and stomach upset at high doses (>600 mg per day).

Vitamin D

Background

Vitamin D is a fat soluble vitamin found in fish liver oil that protects against the complications of diabetes. In addition, vitamin D is necessary for the production of insulin. Antibiotics, laxatives, synthetic fat substitutes, and cholesterol-lowering drugs all interfere with vitamin A and D absorption.

Vitamin D is obtained naturally from two sources, exposure to sunlight and dietary consumption. Vitamin D-3 (cholecalciferol) is the form of vitamin D produced in the skin and consumed in the diet. Vitamin D-2 (ergocalciferol), produced by irradiating fungi, is a much less effective and potentially more toxic source of vitamin D. It is not recommended. In addition to supplementation, sources of vitamin D (other than cow's milk fortified with vitamin D) include fish oil, egg yolks, butter, liver, and some fortified breakfast cereals. Exposure to UV rays found in sunlight enables the body to manufacture vitamin D.

Clinical Studies

Vitamin D, originally believed to influence only calcium absorption and bone density, is now appearing to play an important role in immune system modulation.

Type I Prevention

In a study of more than 12,000 infants in Finland, it was found that vitamin D supplementation was associated with a decreased frequency of Type I diabetes. In fact, regular infants who received the recommend vitamin D supplementation (2,000 IU per day) in the first year of life had an 88% less chance of developing Type I diabetes by age 30 as compared to those infants receiving no supplementation. In addition, children suspected of having rickets during the first year of life (an indicator of low vitamin D status) had a three times higher chance of developing diabetes compared with those children without rickets. The authors conclude that "ensuring adequate vitamin D supplementation for infants could help to reverse the increasing trend in the incidence of type 1 diabetes." It should be noted that the 2,000 IU per day dose recommended is much higher than the North American RDA of 400 IU per day. In this study, infants supplemented with less than 2,000 IU per day did not do as well.

A birth-cohort study undertaken in London over a period of 31years studied the effect of vitamin D in diabetes prevention. Knowing that supplementation with this vitamin reduces the risk of IDDM in animals, the researchers followed more than 10,000 children to measure the effect of vitamin D supplementation in humans. Daily supplementation with 2000 IU of vitamin D (4.5 times the recommended daily allowance) was associated with reduced risk of the development of Type I diabetes.

Insulin Resistance

Low circulating vitamin D levels are also associated with insulin resistance and beta-cell dysfunction, not only in diabetics, but also in healthy young non-diabetic adults. Healthy adults with higher serum vitamin D levels had significantly lower 60-minute, 90-minute, and 120-minute postprandial (after eating) glucose levels than those who were vitamin D deficient. Those with higher vitamin D status also had significantly better insulin sensitivity. The authors noted that, compared with the common oral diabetic pharmaceutical metformin, which improves insulin sensitivity by 13%, higher vitamin D status correlated with a 60% improvement in insulin sensitivity. In addition, a recent clinical trial used 1332 IU per day of vitamin D for only 30 days in 10 women with Type II diabetes. Even this relatively low level of vitamin D supplementation over a short period was shown to improve insulin sensitivity by a remarkable 21%.

Dosage

It is possible that the typical dosage of vitamin D used in supplements, based on the RDA values, is enough to ward off frank deficiency, but falls far short of optimal levels. Full-body exposure to ultraviolet light can produce 10,000 to 25,000 IU of vitamin D-3 per day, much higher than the RDA, and likely more accurately reflecting our needs. It is possible that the majority of studies in adults have used inadequate doses of vitamin D and that is why they may have failed to identify therapeutic benefits from vitamin D supplementation. A more reasonable vitamin D dose for adult studies may be 5,000 to 10,000 IU per day, continued for at least 3 to 4 months until vitamin D levels plateau. Vitamin D therapy should only be undertaken with the guidance of a healthcare practitioner familiar with its use.

Vitamin B-12

Background

Vitamin B-12 plays a critical role in the metabolism of fatty acids that are essential for the maintenance of nerve myelin. It is well known that prolonged B-12 deficiency can lead to nerve degeneration and irreversible neurological damage. Vitamin B-12 is available in three forms: cyanocobalamin, hydrocobalamin, and methylcobalamin. Cyanocobalamin is the most widely available and least expensive form, found in most over-the-counter multivitamins. However, cyanocobalamin is an inactive precursor that must be converted into one of two active metabolites: methylcobalamin and adenosylcobalamin.

Methylcobalamin is essential for folate metabolism and for the formation of choline-containing phospholipids, which are the building blocks of myelin. Adenosylcobalamin is required for the formation of succinyl coenzyme A, the lack of which causes impairment in the formation of neural lipids. Some evidence suggests methylcobalamin is better utilized and retained in the tissues than cyanocobalamin. In addition, many clinicians also claim methylcobalamin is preferred due to improved clinical outcomes.

Clinical Studies

Diabetic Neuropathy

The clinical effectiveness of vitamin B-12 and its active coenzyme for the treatment of diabetic neuropathy was assessed in a meta-analysis of clinical trials to date. Outcomes were measured in these trials based on symptoms or signs, vibration meter detected thresholds of vibration perception, and electrophysiologic measures, such as nerve conduction velocities. Three studies involved the use of vitamin B complex (including B-12) as the active drug and four used methylcobalamin. Both the vitamin B-12 combination and pure methylcobalamin had beneficial effects on somatic symptoms, such as pain and tingling. In three studies, methylcobalamin therapy improved symptoms.

In one study, methylcobalamin was given orally at a dose of 500 mcg, three times per day, to patients with diabetic neuropathy. In this double-blind study, the treatment group showed statistical improvement in the somatic and autonomic symptoms with regression of the signs of diabetic neuropathy. Improvements were noted in burning sensation, pain, numbness, and muscle cramping. The treatment was well tolerated by the patients, and no side effects were observed.

Dosage

The recommended dosage for clinical effect is 5 to 15 mg per day of methylcobalamin, administered orally (sublingually), intramuscularly, or intravenously. Positive clinical results have been reported irrespective of the method of administration. Vitamin B-12 therapy should only be undertaken with the guidance of a healthcare practitioner familiar with its use.

Safety and Side Effects

Methylcobalamin has excellent tolerability and no known toxicity. Alcohol, antibiotics, oral hypoglycemic agents, beta blockers, anti-acid drugs (H2 blockers), oral contraceptives, nicotine, and HIV drugs can all cause vitamin B-12 depletion.

Benfotiamine

Background

Benfotiamine (S-benzoylthiamine-O-monophosphate) is a naturally-occurring fat-soluble form of thiamine (vitamin B-1). However, benfotiamine is believed to be more available to the body than its water soluble counterparts, about five times as great as from conventional thiamine supplements. Benfotiamine is the most potent of the allithiamines, a unique class of thiamine related compounds present in trace quantities in roasted crushed garlic and other members of the *Allium* genus (such as onions, shallots, and leeks).

It has been known for some time that thiamine (vitamin B-1) plays an essential role in the metabolism of glucose, through the actions of its co-enzyme TPP (thiamine pyrophosphate). In the cell, glucose is metabolized in the presence of TPP, and thus TPP is vital to the cell's energy supply and metabolism of glucose. Benfotiamine, acting as a 'super-charged' thiamine, helps maintain healthy cells in the presence of excess blood glucose. It does this through several different mechanisms.

Mechanism of Action

If glucose is maintained at normal levels, excess glucose metabolites do not accumulate within the cell. In the presence of elevated glucose levels, however, the electron transport chain, the final ATP-generating system in the mitochondrion, produces larger than normal amounts of oxygen free-radical superoxide. This excess superoxide inhibits the conversion of glucose to pyruvic acid, resulting in an excess of intermediate metabolites, which trigger several mechanisms that result in potential damage to vascular tissue. Cells particularly vulnerable to this type of damage are found in the retina, kidneys, and nerves.

Benfotiamine has been shown to block three of these mechanisms: the hexosamine pathway, the diaglycerol-protein kinease C pathway, and the formation of advanced glycation end-products (AGE). Benfotiamine does this by stimulating tranketolase, a cellular enzyme essential for maintenance of normal glucose metabolic pathways. Studies done in diabetic rats have shown that benfotiamine counteracts these metabolic abnormalities caused by elevated blood glucose.

Clinical Studies

Advanced Glycation End Product (AGE)

AGE is formed through abnormal linkages between proteins and glucose. This can cause damage to proteins, such as collagen, the major structural protein in connective tissue. This occurs via a reaction similar to the 'browning reaction' that takes place in the cooking and storage of food. High glucose concentrations encourage this, while a return to normal blood glucose levels decrease it.

Because collagen in the body is meant to last, it is more susceptible than other proteins to damage. And because collagen supports a healthy blood vessel wall, damage to collagen compromises vascular function. Furthermore, a number of other potentially harmful events may occur, including immune mediated inflammation that further increases vascular permeability. Accordingly, it is vitally important to support normal glucose metabolic pathways so that formation of AGE is minimized.

Benfotiamine, in the test tube, has been shown to prevent AGE formation in endothelial cells (cells that make up the membranes that line the inner walls of organs and blood vessels) cultured in high glucose. In another study examining the effects of benfotiamine versus water-soluble thiamine, benfotiamine inhibited AGE formation while AGE levels were not significantly altered by thiamine. Of even greater interest, benfotiamine normalized nerve function in the animals. After 6 months of administration, nerve function was normalized by benfotiamine, but not thiamine. In another animal study, benfotiamine was administered to rats with elevated glucose levels, resulting in kidney damage. Benfotiamine improved kidney function and prevented protein leakage into the urine, a commonly used measure of kidney health.

Diabetic Neuropathy

In one trial, 24 people suffering with diabetic neuropathy took either benfotiamine (plus doses of common vitamin B-6 and B-12 similar to those used in mutivitamins) or a placebo, for 12 weeks. The benfotiamine treatment group started with 320 mg of benfotiamine per day for the first 2 weeks, followed by 120 mg for the rest of the trial. Before and after the trial, the function of patients' nerve cells were tested using nerve conduction velocity (NCV) and vibratory perception threshold (when vibrations applied at key nerve sites are first felt). At the end of the trial, the vibration perception threshold had improved by 30% in those who had taken the benfotiamine supplements, while it had worsened in the placebo group. People taking Benfotiamine also experienced a statistically significant improvement in nerve conduction velocity from the feet, while this aspect of nerve function deteriorated in those taking the placebo. No adverse events were reported.

The therapeutic effectiveness of a benfotiamine in diabetic patients suffering from painful peripheral diabetic neuropathy (DNP) was studied in a 6-week open clinical trial. Thirty-six patients were randomly assigned to three groups, each of them comprising 12 participants. One group was given low-dose benfotiamine, while the other groups were given either high-dose benfotiamine plus a standard B vitamin combination or medium-dose benfotiamine plus a standard B vitamin combination. Neuropathy was assessed by five parameters, including the sensation of pain, the vibration sensation, and the current perception threshold.

An overall bneneficial therapeutic effect on the neuropathy status was observed in all three groups during the study, and a significant improvement in most of the parameters studied appeared already at the third week of therapy. The greatest change occurred in the group of patients receiving the high dose. The authors concluded that "benfotiamine is most effective in large doses, although even in smaller daily dosages, either in combination or in monotherapy, it is effective." Furthermore, benfotiamine users have reported 50% to 88% reduction in diabetic nerve pain, depending on the dosage used and the study length, as well as increased ability of the nerves to detect an electrical current.

Retinal Damage

Studies have also begun to document the ability of benfotiamine to protect the tissues of the eye from AGE damage. One study tested the ability of a thiamine/benfotiamine combination to protect the retinas of diabetic rats. The researchers then gave one group of rodents benfotiamine supplements, and left another group unsupplemented. Nine months later, the level of AGE in the retinas of the animals receiving benfotiamine was normal and did not exhibit diabetic retinal damage. Overall, the number of damaged capillaries in the supplemented diabetic animals was indistinguishable from that of their non-diabetic healthy counterparts.

Kidney Damage

Diabetic nephropathy (kidney damage) is a common complication of diabetes associated with a high risk of cardiovascular disease and mortality. In an animal study, therapy with a thiamine/benfotiamine combination countered the accumulation and inhibited the development of nephropathy and strongly inhibited the development of microalbuminuria (protein in the urine due to kidney damage). The authors concluded that "benfotiamine therapy is a potential novel strategy for the prevention of clinical diabetic nephropathy." Further studies are underway to see if benfotiamine can improve kidney function in diabetic animals with pre-existing kidney damage, as it has already been shown to do in the nerves of diabetic animals and humans.

Dosage

Benfotiamine therapy should only be undertaken with the guidance of a healthcare practitioner familiar with its use.

Magnesium

Background

The mineral magnesium functions as an essential cofactor for more than 300 enzymes. Magnesium deficiency has been associated with hypertension, insulin resistance, glucose intolerance, high cholesterol, increased blood clotting, cardiovascular disease, diabetic complications, and complications of pregnancy. Magnesium is one of the more common micronutrient deficiencies in diabetes. Decreased magnesium levels and increased urinary magnesium losses have been documented in both Type I and Type II diabetic patients. In addition, the use of certain medications, including diuretics, can deplete magnesium. Gastrointestinal malabsorption syndromes, low stomach acid (hypochlorydria), diets low in minerals, and alcohol abuse can also cause magnesium depletion.

Clinical Studies

Research has found that low levels of magnesium are associated with poor glycemic control, lower insulin sensitivity, cardiovascular disease, and increased microvascular complications of diabetes. Studies of magnesium supplementation have shown a mild positive effect on insulin sensitivity and triglyceride levels, but mixed results in terms of blood sugar control.

Recent studies have demonstrated that magnesium supplementation may offer protection from the development of NIDDM. One study observed marked magnesium deficiency in 11 well-controlled Type II diabetics; supplementation over 8 weeks significantly raised free intracellular magnesium in the subjects. The protective aspect of magnesium was isolated by another study that examined the effect of magnesium supplementation on obese rats over a period of 6 weeks. By the end of the study period, all of the control animals became diabetic, while only one of the eight rats in the supplementation group developed the disease. By preventing deterioration of glucose tolerance, magnesium may thus delay or prevent Type II diabetes.

Dosage

The America Diabetic Association recommends assessment of magnesium status in patients at risk for deficiency and supplementation for deficiencies. Research suggests that relatively high doses of magnesium for 3 months, followed by lower daily supplements, are needed to restore and maintain magnesium in people with diabetes. Doses of 300 to 600 mg per day of magnesium citrate are appropriate for patients with normal kidney function. Good dietary sources include whole grains, leafy green vegetables, legumes, nuts, and fish. Diets high in saturated fat, sugar, fructose, caffeine, and alcohol may increase magnesium requirements. Magnesium therapy should only be undertaken with the guidance of a healthcare practitioner familiar with its use.

Vitamin B-3 (Niacin or Niacinamide)

Background

Vitamin B-3 (also known as niacin or niacinamide) is an essential nutrient for fat, carbohydrate, and cholesterol metabolism. It is also a component of glucose tolerance factor. Food sources of vitamin B-3 include legumes, milk, organ meats, liver, eggs, fish, peanuts and whole grains.

Clinical Studies

Type I Prevention

Supplementation with niacinamide (also called nicotinamide) has been shown in both animal and human studies to offer protection from the development of Type I diabetes. There have been six clinical, double-blind, placebo-controlled studies performed on the use of niacinamide on patients suffering from Type I diabetes within 5 years of their diagnosis. Of these six studies, three have demonstrated a positive effect in promoting remission, lowering insulin requirements, and increasing beta cell function (the cells that make insulin). Some of the recently diagnosed Type I patients were able to go into complete remission with niacinamide. The most positive results were achieved in subjects who were older and had higher fasting C-peptide levels.

Theoretically, niacinamide acts as an antioxidant that modulates the immune system's attack on the pancreatic beta cells. In recent onset Type I diabetes, niacinamide has been shown to slow the destruction of the beta cells in the pancreas, preserving, increasing, and, in some cases, restoring the function of the beta cells. Baseline C-peptide, a measure of endogenous insulin preservation and Hb1ac, can be maintained when niacinamide is added to insulin therapy. The mechanism of action is thought to be an inhibition of macrophage and interleukin-1 mediated beta cell damage and inhibition of nitric oxide production, along with its antioxidant activity.

Dosage

A dosage of 25 mg per kg of body weight is commonly used. Niacinamide therapy should only be undertaken with the guidance of a healthcare practitioner familiar with its use.

Other Recommended Supplements

Vitamin A

Diabetics do not usually do well in converting the carotenes into vitamin A, so supplementation is recommended. Vitamin A is an antioxidant that also stimulates the secretion of gastric juices for digesting protein and assimilating calcium, required for proper growth.

The fat-soluble form of vitamin A is found in butter fat (especially from pasture-fed animals), egg yolks, liver, organ meats, seafood, and fish liver oil. Although carotenes are water soluble precursors to vitamin A, on food labels they may be listed as vitamin A. This can be misleading.

Vitamin B-6

Vitamin B-6 deficiencies have been linked to diabetes, as well as many other chronic disorders. Production of pancreatic enzymes, required for proper digestion and absorption of other nutrients, requires vitamin B-6 and zinc.

Vitamin B-6 is one of the most difficult nutrients to obtain in the North American diet because it is found mainly in raw animal food. Some health food stores carry naturally cured cheese made from raw milk, a good source for B-6 for people who do not have a dairy allergy or sensitivity. Imported cheese if labeled "milk" or "fresh milk" is usually a cheese made from raw milk.

Sodium

Salt (sodium chloride) is necessary for the production of hydrochloric acid, essential for good digestion. It is also necessary for proper functioning of the adrenal glands. Unprocessed sea salt (pink, beige, or grey in color) is far better than processed salt (sea salt or not) and iodized salt. All processed salts are practically devoid of trace minerals, which are found in unprocessed sea salt. Trace minerals are also found in homemade bone broths, red meats, shellfish, extra virgin olive oil, organ meats, nutritional yeasts, and molasses.

Borage, Black Currant, and Evening Primrose Oil

These oils are recommended because they are high in GLA, crucial for people suffering from diabetes, and supply some of the enzymes missing in the modern diet.

Cod Liver Oil and Fish Oils

These oils provide the essential vitamins A and D. They play a large role in helping to regulate blood sugar levels through lowering insulin resistance. They are best taken in the winter months, but may be taken year round in flavored liquid or capsule form.

Powdered Greens

Powder green foods contain many essential nutrients and chlorophyll for cell renewal. Spirulina is also considered to help control blood sugar levels.

Antioxidants

High doses of a variety of antioxidants help lessen the formation of damaging free radicals. It is a good idea to include various forms of antioxidants in the diet because they work best together. Good antioxidants include vitamin C (calcium ascorbate), vitamin E, pycnogenol, grapeseed extract, selenium, vitamin A, and alpha-lipoic acid (ALA). ALA not only helps balance blood sugar levels, prevent neuropathy, and repair nerve damage, it also helps 'neutralize' the small amount of free radicals created with other antioxidants. Fresh juices, best made from green vegetables for people with diabetes, act as a form of antioxidant with the end product of harmless hydrogen. Remember to include some good fat or oil to aid the absorption of the minerals from these health-giving drinks.

Probiotics

Probiotics need to be supplemented regularly to aid digestion and absorption, especially if lacto-fermented foods are not consumed or antibiotics are used. Probiotics also help to treat and prevent opportunistic infections that diabetics are susceptible to, such as *Candida albicans*.

BOTANICAL MEDICINE THERAPY

More than half of the population of North America suffers from a chronic disease, such as arthritis, allergies, high blood pressure, depression, chronic pain, digestive problems, or diabetes. Conventional pharmaceutical medicine often cannot provide a satisfactory solution or merely manages the symptoms of these diseases while creating uncomfortable and even debilitating side effects. As a result, people are increasingly looking to alternative therapies, such as homeopathic medicine, traditional Asian medicine, and botanical medicine to improve their quality of life.

One major criticism of these alternative therapies is that they are "unproven" and potentially "unsafe." This criticism is rarely justified. In most cases, evidence does exist in various forms – clinical trials, case studies, anecdotal evidence, and traditional knowledge. For example, ample trials have been run on specific medicinal herbs to show their efficacy in preventing, treating, and, in some cases, reversing diabetes and the complications of diabetes. Many medicinal herbs have properties not unlike the pharmaceutical drugs used in managing diabetes.

Botanicals for Type II Diabetes

Several herbs have been demonstrated in clinical studies to be effective for treating Type II diabetes and supporting the glands and organs of the endocrine system. For many years, physicians have been successfully using these herbs to reduce insulin levels. In fact, the herb goat's rue (*Galega officinalis*) is the original source of the chemical compounds known as biguanides, derivatives of which are still the main type of oral hypoglycemic used today. Herbal treatments as opposed to "mono" drug therapy seem to work in a number of synergistic ways, slowing glucose release into the blood after meals, supporting pancreatic islet cell function, protecting nerve and blood vessel cells from oxidative damage, and improving insulin sensitivity.

Among the most clinically effective herbs for treating Type II diabetes are milk thistle (*Silybum marianum*), gymnema (*Gymnema sylvestre*), nopal (*Nopal opuntia spp.*), jambul (*Syzygium jambolana*), globe artichoke (*Cynara scolymus* L.) and devil's club (*Oplopanax horridus*). Monographs describing their pharmacology and clinical applications are provided here.

Milk Thistle (Silybum marianum)

Background

Silybum marianum is currently the most researched herb in the treatment of liver disease (with over 450 published peer review papers). The active constituent of silybum is silymarin, a mixture of flavonolignans consisting chiefly of silibin, silidianin, and silichristine. Silibin is the most active of the three and is largely responsible for the benefits attributed to the silymarin complex.

Pharmacology

Silybum exerts a protective and restorative effect on the liver. The hepato-protective effects include antioxidation, antilipid peroxidation, enhanced detoxification, and protection against glutathione depletion. Silybum inhibits the enzyme lipoxygenase, thereby inhibiting the formation of the hepato-destructive leukotrienes. In damaged livers, silymarin has been shown to increase protein synthesis, which might account for its hepatorestorative action. Silymarin has been shown in animal studies to possess antifibrotic activity. Animal and in-vitro studies have shown sily-bum to possess antidiabetic, antitumor, antiatherosclerotic, and anti-nephrotoxic activity.

Clinical Studies

A number of studies have shown that silymarin may be valuable in the prophylaxis and treatment of diabetes and its complications.

Blood Sugar and Insulin Control

Treatment with the milk thistle flavonoid silymarin resulted in lowered, fasting blood glucose levels, mean daily blood glucose levels, daily gluco-suria, and HbA1c. In addition, fasting insulin levels and mean exogenous insulin requirements were reduced. Silymarin may reduce the lipo-perox-idation of cell membranes and insulin resistance, significantly decreasing endogenous insulin overproduction and the need for exogenous insulin administration.

Silymarin also decreased basal and glucagon-stimulated C-peptide levels. In treatment with silibin, there was a highly significant reduction in RBC sorbitol, though no effect on fasting blood glucose, and an improved nerve conduction velocity, though not statistically significant. Silibin may be a potent aldose reductase inhibitor and may be valuable in the prophy-laxis and treatment of diabetic complications. In the treatment of rats, sili-bin prevented the onset of diabetic neuropathy, possibly by inhibiting excessive protein mono-ADP-ribosylation.

Silymarin may also reduce lipo-oxidation of hepatic cell membranes and help reverse insulin resistance. Silibin, which is one of the three flavolignans in silymarin, was studied on patients with NIDDM. The sor-bitol red blood cell (RBC) level for 14 patients with NIDDM averaged 72.5 mmol/g; this was two times higher than the control group that didn't have diabetes. In this study, 231 mg of silibin was administered for 4 weeks to the NIDDM patients: their sorbitol RBC level dropped to 39.53 mmol/g. The study also found slightly improved nerve conduction velocity in the silibin group. Silibin, a potent aldose reductase inhibitor, is valuable in the prophylaxis and prevention of complications in diabetes.

The adrenal gland has a function in the regulation of insulin called the Somogyi phenomenon. In response to hypoglycemia, epinephrine, norepinephrine, and cortisol are secreted by the adrenal gland. In diabetic rats, a short-term diabetic state lowered the activity of their adrenal cortex. Thus, subclinical adrenal hypofunction should be assessed in NIDDM patients.

Diabetic Neuropathy

Milk thistle is also effective in the treatment of neuropathy. Silibin is a flavonoid, which is a mono-adenoid di-phosphate-lipoxyl-transferase inhibitor. It helps to prevent protein ADP ribosylation. ADP ribosylation causes an increase in P-like substance that, in turn, causes an immunoreactivity level that is found in diabetic neuropathy. In the treatment of diabetic rats, silibin was found to prevent the increase of ADP ribosylation in Schwann cells.

Secondary Diabetes

Milk thistle has been shown to be an effective treatment for patients with diabetes secondary to cirrhosis. In a trial done in Italy, 30 diabetic patients were given a regime of conventional therapy and 600 mg daily of silymarin, while 30 other patients were given only conventional therapy. After 4 months, the group who using 600 mg daily of silymarin had decreased fasting glucose levels, decreased glucosuria, decreased HbA1c values, and decreased fasting insulin levels, with a decreased exogenous insulin requirement. The control group had increased insulin levels after the study and stabilization of exogenous insulin needs. This study demonstrated that silymarin decreased endogenous insulin overproduction and decreased exogenous insulin requirements in patients with liver disease. Milk thistle stimulates protein synthesis, resulting in the regeneration of hepatic cells and new liver tissue.

Contraindications

Silybum is virtually free of toxicity. In animals, silymarin was shown to be non-toxic when administered at high doses for short periods. Long-term administration to rats also demonstrated an absence of toxicity. Silybum can stimulate liver and gallbladder activity and can therefore produce a transient laxative effect. Mild allergic reactions have been noted.

Dosage

Since silymarin is not water soluble, administration as an infusion is not recommended. The standard dose of silybum is based on its silymarin content (70 to 210 mg capsules three times daily). A higher dosage will likely yield better results. Several animal and human studies have shown that silymarin bound to phosphatidylcholine yields better absorption and clinical effect (dose 100 to 200 mg twice daily).

Gymnema (Gymnema sylvestre)

Background

Gymnema sylvestre is a member of the Asclepiadaceae family. It has been used in Ayurvedic medicine to treat madhu meha or "honey urine." Gymnema came to be known as gurmar or the "destroyer of sugar" because Ayurvedic physicians observed that chewing a few leaves suppressed the taste of sugar. It has been used in India for the treatment of diabetes for 2,000 years.

The medicinally active parts of the plant are the leaves and the roots. Plant constituents include two resins (one soluble in alcohol), gymnemic acids, saponins, stigmasterol, quercitol, and the amino acid derivatives betaine, choline, and trimethylamine.

Pharmacology

The important active ingredient in *Gymnema sylvestre* is an organic acid called gymnemic acid. This is a triterpene glycoside that suppresses sweetness in humans. From this glycosidic fraction, six triterpene glycosides – gymnemosides a, b, c, d, e, and f – were isolated. There are four triterpenoid saponins and six known gymnemic acids found in *G. sylvestre*. However, the principal constituents are gymnemic acid and gymnemasaponin. Gurmarin is a polypeptide isolated from the leaves that consists of 35 amino acid residues, including three intramolecular disulfide bonds. It has a molecular weight of 4,000 and is inhibitory to neural responses to sweet taste stimuli.

Mechanism of Action

Gymnema sylvestre is a stomachic, diuretic, refrigerant, astringent, and tonic. Its antidiabetic activity is due to a combination of mechanisms. Recent pharmacological studies have shown that gymnema acts on both the taste buds in the oral mucosa and the absorptive surface to the intestines.

The structure of the taste buds that detect sugar in the mouth is similar to the structure of the tissue that absorbs sugar in the intestines. The active ingredient, gymnemic acid, acts on both these sites.

Gymnemic acid is made up of molecules whose atom arrangement is similar to that of glucose molecules. Those molecules fill the receptor locations on the taste buds for a period of 1 to 2 hours, thereby preventing the taste buds from being activated by any sugar molecule present in food. Similarly, the glucose-like molecules in the gymnemic acid fill the receptor locations in the absorptive external layers of the intestine, thereby preventing the intestine from absorbing the sugar molecules. Therefore, gymnemic acids from the leaves suppress the elevation of blood glucose level by inhibiting glucose uptake in the intestines. The leaves also contain chlorophyll, xanthophylls, carotene, phytol, and lime salts. *Gymnema sylvestre* has also been found to reduce the bitter taste of certain foods.

Gymnema increases the activity of enzymes responsible for glucose uptake and utilization, and inhibits peripheral utilization of glucose by somatotrophin and corticotrophin. Extracts of this plant have also been found to inhibit epinephrine-induced hyperglycemia. Gymnema has even been shown to regenerate insulin-producing beta cells of the pancreas, leading to an enhancement in the production of endogenous insulin, further controlling blood sugar. Gymnema inhibits adrenocortical activity and prevents the normal hyperglycemic response of the anterior pituitary gland, which acts in turn by inhibiting peripheral glucose metabolism induced by somatotropin and corticotropin hormones. The extracts from gymnema leaves have been shown to suppress the intestinal smooth muscle contraction, decrease oxygen consumption, inhibit the glucose evoked-transmural potential, and prevent increased blood glucose levels. Studies indicate gymnema inhibits the increase in the blood glucose level by interfering with the intestinal glucose absorption process.

Gymnema is antiviral. It increases oxygen uptake, blood pressure, and secretions of liver and pancreas. The leaves have been found to stimulate the heart, uterus, and circulatory system. It raises urine output. As an agent to promote weight loss, gymnema may help control appetite and carbohydrate cravings.

Gymnema increases the blood's capacity to take up oxygen, resulting in higher physical and mental performance and increased energy levels. This is beneficial for keeping in shape and staying active. The leaves are used for stomach ailments, constipation, water retention, and liver disease. The leaves are also noted for lowering serum cholesterol and triglycerides.

Clinical Studies
Recent clinical trials have shown that *Gymnema sylvestre* is useful for treating both insulin-dependent diabetes mellitus (IDDM) and non-insulin dependent diabetes mellitus (NIDDM).

Blood Sugar and Insulin Control
The first scientific confirmation of gymnema's use in diabetes came almost 70 years ago when it was demonstrated that the leaves reduced urine glucose in diabetics. Four years later, it was shown that gymnema had a blood glucose lowering effect when there was residual pancreatic function, but was without effect in animals lacking pancreatic function, suggesting a direct effect on the pancreas.

Another study showed that in diabetic rats, fasting blood glucose levels returned to normal after 60 days of gymnema with oral administration. The therapy led to a rise in serum insulin to levels closer to normal fasting levels. In diabetic rat pancreas, gymnema was able to double the islet number and beta cell number.

In 1981, it was demonstrated that oral administration of the dried leaves of gymnema brings down blood glucose and raises serum insulin levels. In 1988, a study showed a normalization of glycosylated hemoglobin and plasma proteins (indicators of long term glucose control) from gymnema administration. In 1990, it was shown that administration of gymnema extract to diabetic animals was accompanied by a regeneration of beta cells in the pancreas. This brought about glucose homeostasis through increased serum insulin levels provided by repair/regeneration of the pancreas.

A study was conducted on both Type I and II diabetics given a standardized gymnema extract, from the leaves, for a period of 2 years. Twenty-seven patients with IDDM who were on insulin therapy were administered 400 mg per day of gymnema for 6 to 30 months. Insulin requirements were decreased by about one-half and the average blood glucose decreased from 232 mg/dL to 152 mg/dL. Glycosylated plasma protein levels also decreased. Gymnema appeared to enhance endogenous insulin by regeneration of the residual beta cells in IDDM. Serum lipids also returned to normal levels with gymnema therapy, which may help prevent cardiovascular disease. Most impressively, an increase in C-peptide levels were found, which is a strong indication of restoration of insulin production.

Dr Baskaran and Dr Ahamath, at the Department of Biochemistry, Post-Graduate Institute of Basic Medical Sciences in Madras, India, investigated the therapeutic properties of an extract from the leaves of *Gymnema sylvestre* in controlling hyperglycemia in 22 Type II diabetic patients on conventional oral anti-hyperglycemic agents. *Gymnema sylvestre* (400 mg per day) was administered for 18 to 20 months as a supplement to the conventional oral drugs. During supplementation, the patients showed a significant reduction in blood glucose, glycosylated hemoglobin, and glycosylated plasma proteins. Conventional drug dosage could be decreased. Five of the 22 diabetic patients were able to discontinue their conventional drug and maintain their blood glucose homeostasis with *Gymnema sylvestre* alone. These data suggest that the beta cells may be regenerated/repaired in Type II diabetic patients on *Gymnema sylvestre* supplementation. This is supported by the appearance of raised insulin levels in the serum of patients after gymnema supplementation. Additionally, gymnema significantly improved cholesterol, triglyceride, and free fatty acid levels that were elevated.

Adaptogenic Effect
Some authors are speaking of the "adaptogenic" nature of gymnema, since it increases the body's ability to adapt to the presence of sugar. The increase in longevity noted above was ascribed to "cardiotonic and adaptogenic characteristics produced by increasing resistance and immunity in diabetic animals." To be a true adaptogen, it would need to "normalize" function, not just prolong life. Recently, researchers have reported gymnema prevents death due to hypoglycemia in rats injected with beryllium nitrate. That gymnema prevents both rises and falls in blood sugar and causes no significant change in normal blood sugar levels appears to be in full harmony with the concept of an adaptogen.

In other animal studies, gymnema has been found to double the number of insulin-secreting beta cells in the pancreas and return blood sugar to almost normal. Most cases have shown it to lower blood sugar to normal levels and not to a point below normal, as seen with many other antidiabetic drugs. However, studies conducted in India as early as 1930 showed that the leaves could cause hypoglycemia in experimental animals.

The anti-sweet peptide, gurmarin, purified from the leaves of *Gymnema sylvestre*, is highly specific to sweet taste so that responses to various sweeteners are all suppressed. Gurmarin acts on the apical side of the taste cell, possibly by binding to the sweet taste receptor protein.

In a very thorough animal study, gymnema greatly reduced the blood glucose levels in alloxan-induced diabetic rabbits. It was thought gymnema effects were mediated through stimulation of insulin release resembling what was observed with sulfonylureas, or through inhibition of intestinal absorption of glucose as observed with the biguanides, or through stimulation of one of the insulinogenic signals promoting insulin release.

Gymnema reversed the glycogen and protein depletions and lipid accumulation in the diabetic animals. The theory that gymnema works by increasing the levels of circulating insulin was supported by observations of altered enzyme activities in the liver, kidney, and muscles. Most of the insulin-dependent enzymes (hexokinase, glycogen synthetase, glyceraldehyde-3-phosphate dehydrogrenase, and glucose-6-phosphate dehydrogenase) were significantly more active in the gymnema-treated animals than in control diabetic animals. It also increased the activity of enzymes affecting the utilization of glucose by insulin-dependent pathways: phosphorylase, gluconeogenic enzymes, and sorbitol dehydrogenase. Pathological changes in liver and kidney were reversed by the treatment. The study reports in great detail findings supporting the notion that gymnema corrects the metabolic derangements in diabetic rabbit liver, kidney, and muscle tissues.

Other studies have found similar normalizing effects of various enzymes and chemicals of the kidney, heart, liver and brain, including hexuronic acid, hexoses, hexosamines, non-amino polysaccharides, hyaluronic acid, heparin sulfate, chondroitin sulfates, and sialic acid.

In another study utilizing alloxan diabetic rabbits and one human patient, gymnema brought down the fasting blood glucose levels, together with serum cholesterol and triglyceride levels, while improving serum protein levels. The hypoglycemic action took several weeks to develop. Oral administration in normal rats apparently has no significant effect, but only in rats made hyperglycemic experimentally (alloxan, anterior pituitary-treated, tolbutamide, adrenaline).

While gymnema does not lower blood sugar levels in normal subjects, it does appear to prevent a rise in blood sugar levels in normal subjects. This result has been attributed to a pancreotropic effect due to sensitization of beta cells of islets of Langerhans for secreting larger amounts of insulin in response to glucose. In addition, it markedly inhibited somatotropin- and corticotropin-induced elevations in blood sugar levels.

An interesting finding in clinical tests showed that healthy people with normal insulin levels showed no lowering of blood sugar levels or hypoglycemic effects after taking the herb.

Dosage

Gymnema sylvestre in tea form offers the best results. It has been determined that a daily dose of 200 mg is optimal in order to utilize its effectiveness in the area of weight management. The typical therapeutic dose (for treatment of hyperglycemia), standardized to contain 24% gymnemic acids, is 400 to 600 mg daily. In adult-onset diabetics, ongoing use for periods as long as 18 to 24 months has proven successful. In reducing the symptoms of glycosuria, the dried leaves are used in daily doses of 3 to 4 grams for 3 to 4 months. Because it acts gradually, gymnema extract should be consumed regularly with meals for several days or weeks and can be taken for months or years with no significant side effects.

Drug Interactions

Patients taking gymnema may require dosage adjustments of other antidiabetic drugs. However, in some cases, it may make the treatment more effective. Some patients do develop hypoglycemia when taking gymnema along with other medications. This is because improved insulin production and release during gymnema therapy may decrease the need for other medication and thus lower blood glucose levels, unless the dosage of conventional oral medication or insulin is lowered.

Some of the effects of gymnema may be enhanced by MAOI antidepressant medications, fenfluramine, salicylates, and tetracyclines. Its actions may even be decreased by concomitant use of oral contraceptives, epinephrine, phenothiazines, marijuana, and thyroid hormones. Gymnema has diuretic action that increases the renal excretion of sodium and chloride, and may potentiate the hyperglycemic and hyperuremic effects of glucose elevating agents. Patients using diuretics may require dosage adjustments of antidiabetic drugs.

Certain botanical medications, including antidepressants (St. John's wort) and salicylates (white willow and aspirin), can enhance the blood sugar-lowering effects of *Gymnema sylvestre*, whereas certain stimulants, such as ephedra (Ma Huang), may reduce its effectiveness. The antidiabetic ability of this herb may be decreased by concomitant use of acetazolamide, oral contraceptives, corticosteroids, dextrothyroxine, epinephrine, ethanol, glucagon, guanethidine, and marijuana. The antidiabetic effects may also be decreased when used in conjunction with phenothiazines, rifampin, thiazide diuretics, and thyroid hormones.

The antidiabetic action of gymnema may be enhanced when it is used with allopurinol, anabolic steroids, chloramphenicol, clofibrate, fenfluramine, guanethidine, MAOI, phenylbutazone, probenecid, and phenyramidol. This action of gymnema may also be enhanced when used in conjunction with salicylates, sulfinpyrazone, sulfonamides, and tetracyclines. The ability of gymnema to increase insulin production and secretion may be antagonized by heparin.

Adverse Reactions

At typical recommended doses, dietary supplements containing gymnema are not associated with significant adverse side effects. Mild gastrointestinal upset may occur if gymnema is taken on an empty stomach; therefore, consumption with meals is recommended. Caution is urged, however, with extremely high doses, which may have the potential to induce hypoglycemia in susceptible individuals. It can also alter the bitter and sweet taste sensation.

Nopal (Nopal opuntia spp)

Background

Also known as prickly pear and beaver tail, nopal is native to arid and semi-arid areas of North America and South America. Nopal has no leaves, except at the start of new growth. These leaves are actually stems called cladodes that grow one on top of another in an irregular, beavertail shaped pattern. It has spiny, thickened stems that form the plant and produce yellow, orange, and red rose-like flowers in the spring. These flowers mature into prickly pears, which are yellow, orange, red, or purple. The fruits are sweet, with numerous hard seeds. They survive under a variety of severe climates and can regenerate themselves. The pads are skinned, diced, and prepared in Mexican salads and tacos.

Pharmacology

The mechanism of nopal is unknown; however, one study suggested it was associated with gastric distension and enterohormones. In another study, the mechanisms of cellular sensitivity to insulin in addition to dietary fiber was suspected, because blood sugar was reduced in the absence of an oral carbohydrate load; this study further showed that serum insulin concentration diminished after taking nopal, thus ruling out an enhancement of insulin release. A different study ruled out the involvement of insulin antagonist hormones, like glucagon, cortisol, and growth hormone.

Nopal contains vitamin B, vitamin C, calcium, iron, potassium, B-carotene, and the carbohydrates: hexoses, pentoses, cellulose hemicellulose, and mucilage. Nopal is high in fiber, protein, and amino acid composition.

Clinical Applications

Nopal is hypoglycemic, hypolipidemic, antimicrobial, vulnerary, demulcent, and nutritive. It is used for gastritis and peptic ulcers, high cholesterol, enlargement of the prostate gland, and diabetes. Externally, it is used for dry, itchy scalp and wound healing.

In patients with NIDDM, studies have shown that nopal significantly reduced glucose and fasting insulin serum concentrations. Nopal lowered blood sugar when orally administered to animals with induced states of moderate hyperglycemia. Nopal does not significantly modify fasting glucose levels and insulin serum concentrations in healthy individuals; however, it reduces the elevation of glucose and insulin serum concentrations after an oral glucose load.

In addition to the diabetic effect, nopal reduced LDL cholesterol, total cholesterol, and triglycerides when taken before each meal for 10 days. The triglyceride levels were decreased in obese and diabetic patients, but not in healthy subjects with low triglyceride levels.

Drug Interactions

Since nopal does not tend to lower blood sugar levels if they are normal, it is highly unlikely that hypoglycemia might occur with nopal alone; however, hypoglycemic agents might need to be decreased if used in combination with nopal.

Dosage

Recommended dose is 100 g of nopal stems grilled or 3 tablespoons of prickly pear fruit concentrate daily.

Jambul (Syzygium jambolana)

Background

Jambul is native to southern Asia, India, Indonesia, and Australia. The seed is hard, oval, and red brown to brown. Jambul fruit is eaten as a preserve; it tastes faintly astringent and aromatic, like a ripe apricot. The fruit contains volatile oil, fixed oil, resin, tannins, and gallic acid, as well as phenols, tannins, triterpenoids, glycosides, volatile oils, and alkaloids (jambosine).

Pharmacology

Animal studies have shown a pronounced hypoglycemic effect. It also has an anti-inflammatory effect in animals. The method of action may be independent of pancreatic function; it may alter the conversion of carbohydrates to glucose.

Clinical Applications

Jambul is astringent, carminative, hypoglycemic, antispasmodic, and stomatic. The seed is considered to be one of the most powerful hypoglycemic agents in the Ayurvedic repertory. In India, as little as 1 teaspoon per day of ground seed was a traditional treatment for NIDDM. Externally, the astringent action is useful for nosebleeds and wounds.

Dosage

Recommended dose is 0.3-2 g infusion, 1:1 in 25% alcohol, 2-4 ml t.i.d.

Globe Artichoke (Cynara scolymus L.)

Background

Globe artichoke is a perennial plant found in the Mediterranean region and South America.

Pharmacology

Constituents of the flower heads are 12% sugar (inulin), 3% protein, tannin, cynarin, vitamins A, B1, B2, B3, C, caffeic acid, flavonoids (rutin), and sesquiterpenes lactones.

The inulin in globe artichoke is a polymer of fructose that is not digested and does not increase blood sugar. It decreases postprandial hyperglycemia. In research, 20 g caused only a mild rise in blood sugar, which was significantly lower than the same dose of fructose. Inulin, which may be broken down to fructose in cold weather or winter months and converted back in summer months, activates the complement pathway and promotes chemotaxis of neutrophils, monocytes, and eosinophils. It also may stimulate interferon. Cynarin (15% content in roots) stimulates bile and has a direct effect on liver function. It is broken down into caffeic acids, which act on the liver. The bitters may also contain small amount of caffeic acid.

Clinical Applications

Traditionally, globe artichoke was used for arteriosclerosis, hyperlipidemia, and diabetes. In France, it was used for gallstones, obesity, and rheumatism. Globe artichoke is indicated for arteriosclerosis, jaundice, dyspepsia, anorexia, liver insufficiency, chronic albuminuria, post-operative anemia, gallbladder, and biliary disease, chronic liver disease and impairment, and kidney disease. It increases excretion and decreases synthesis of total cholesterol. It helps to prevent gallstone formation.

Globe artichoke is also attributed with tonic, choleretic, cholagogue, diuretic, laxative, antigalactic, alterative, and aphrodisiac qualities. It stimulates liver cells to regenerate and is also hepato-protective. It supports the kidneys and has a hypoglycemic effect in diabetes.

Contraindications

Theoretically, globe artichoke is contraindicated for biliary tree blockage and colic, which may be due to active gallstones.

Dosage

Recommended dose is 1-4 g dried leaves three times daily, or up to 15-30 ml of tincture per day.

Devil's Club (Oplopanax horridus)

Background

Devil's club constituents possibly include saponins and inulin. In North America, Southwest natives believed regular use could prevent cancer.

Clinical Studies

Pharmacology

Devil's club attracted medical attention in 1938 when Dr Brocklesby (MD) discovered that a patient was stabilizing diabetes with an infusion of devil's club. In lab tests conducted by Brocklesby and Large in 1938, devil's club showed no apparent toxicity. The hypoglycemic effect of devil's club extract is especially significant in view of the longstanding controversy over the use and toxicity of present antidiabetic drugs. Experiments done on rabbits demonstrated that an extract of the herb would substantially reduce blood sugar without any toxic side effects.

Devil's club is used for arthritis, rheumatism, stomach pains, constipation, and especially for the prevention and treatment of diabetes. The bark can be burnt and applied to cuts. A paste can be made out of the root powder and applied as a poultice to decrease pain and swelling from insect bites and stings.

Dosage

Recommended dose is 1-2 g, three times daily.

Clinical Studies: Botanical Combination Therapy

Certain botanicals used in combination have proven to be effective in treating dysglycemia. In this trial, jambul, nopal, globe artichoke, milk thistle, and devil's club were combined.

Methods: Starting in September 1998, we tested a herbal formula on 20 patients suffering from dysglycemia. The encapsulated formula contained the herbs jambul, devil's club, milk thistle, nopal, and globe artichoke, which was referred to as the Jambul combo. Ten patients with NIDDM were given the formula for a 3-month period. One patient with Type I/II was given the herbs for 3 months. One patient with Type I was given the formula for a 3-month period. One patient with hyperinsulinemia was given the herbs for 3 months, and seven patients with sub-clinical hypoglycemia were given the formula for 6 weeks.

Most participants in the study were also taking pharmacological agents. One NIDDM patient and the hypoglycemia patients were not on any pharmaceutical treatments during the study period.

Criteria: Five people were disqualified after the study for not matching the above criteria. Patients who had a weight change of more than 5 pounds within the 3 months were not included in the final data. Patients who had made dietary, lifestyle, and/or prescription drug changes were also disregarded. Patients who had not taken prescribed herbal dosages were disqualified at the end of the study.

Setting: Five outpatient clinics in Canada, the United States, and India, supervised by medical doctors and licensed naturopathic physicians.

Results:
Patient #1
Condition: Diabetes Type II
Onset of Diabetes: 6 years
Pharmacological Treatment: Metformin 500 mg b.i.d. and Diamicron 160 mg b.i.d. The patient had poor blood sugar control with the medicine before the study. She had taken chromium with little result.
Natural Medicine: Jambul combo three pills t.i.d.
Fasting Blood Sugar and Other Indications:
Average for the week of May 23, 1999 was about 16 mmol/L (288 mg/dL).
Average on June 1st was 15.9 mmol/L (286 mg/dL).
Average on June 7th was 13.6 mmol/L (245 mg/dL).
Average on June 14th was 12.2 mmol/L (220 mg/dL).
Average on June 21 was 12.3 mmol/L (221 mg/dL).
Average on June 27 was 9.5 mmol/L (171 mg/dL).

After 3 months, the patient averaged about 11.2mmol/L (201.6mg/dL). She had noticed effects of the treatment within 2 weeks. Her glycosylated hemoglobin HbA1c value was 10.2%, and after 3 months of treatment was 9.8%. She maintained her pharmacological treatment during the study.

Patient #2

Condition: Diabetes Type II

Onset of Diabetes: 10 years

Pharmacological Treatment: For NIDDM, Humulin 44 AM and PM, Toronto AM, and six units of insulin PM. History of diabetic treatment before the study was 9 years of oral hypoglycemics and 1 year of insulin. During this time the patient developed hypertension, angina, chronic renal failure (60% failure in both kidneys).

Natural Medicine: Jambul combo one pill t.i.d., and 600 mcg of chromium. A goldenrod tincture was prescribed for kidney support.

Fasting Blood Sugar and Other Indications: Fasting blood sugar level before the study was 2.2 mmol/L (220mg/dL). After 3 months, levels dropped to 8.8 mmol/L (158 mg/dL). Glycosylated hemoglobin was 7.9% before the study and after 3 months was 7.8%. Blood sugar levels were reduced while she decreased the dosage of her pharmaceutical drugs. Patient's insulin levels lowered to 42 Humulin and 4 Toronto. After the study, the patient needed three injections daily, instead of the five, as needed previously. The patient also experienced less back pain, which allowed her to start walking again, something she was unable to do before due to the severity of pain caused by her kidney damage. Her creatinine level decreased from 138 to 115 mmol/L.

Patient #3

Condition: Diabetes Type II

Onset of Diabetes: 25 years

Pharmacological Treatment: For NIDDM, Metformin 500 mg, 2 pills b.i.d., Glyburide 5 mg, b.i.d. These pharmaceutical drugs were discontinued upon starting the study. This patient was able to achieve normal blood sugar levels while on the drugs. However, due to the severe side effects of the pharmaceutical agents, specifically leg edema and flu like symptoms, she had discontinued the drugs.

Natural Medicine: Jambul combo three pills t.i.d.

Fasting Blood Sugar/Other indications: Fasting blood sugar on waking averaged around 15 mmol/L (270 mg/dL). She maintained this level for several weeks without the use of any treatment. Within several days of taking the herbs, her fasting blood sugar level went down to 9 mmol/L (162mg/dL). She had no leg edema or flu-like symptoms. Glycosylated hemoglobin was normal before the study, and after, it was 7.0%. The patient was near the American Diabetic Association recommendation target range of glycosylated hemoglobin without using the pharmacological agents sulfonylurea and biguanide due to her use of Jambul combo. The patient had no kidney pain at the end of the study.

Patient #4
Condition: Diabetes Type II
Onset of Diabetes: 25 years
Pharmacological Treatment: For NIDDM, insulin for the past 25 years.
Natural Medicine: Jambul combo, two pills b.i.d., and 400 mg of lipoic acid and golden rod tincture for kidney support. (Note at this dose, lipoic acid has no effect on fasting blood sugar levels.)
Fasting Blood Sugar/Other Indications: Fasting blood sugar levels averaged around 158 mg/dL (8.8 mmol/L). After 3 months, levels averaged around 100 mg/dL (5.56 mmol/L), which is a completely normal blood sugar level. Her diabetic nephropathy had decreased and the edema and blood streaks in her legs were gone at the end of this study. Exogenous insulin requirements decreased by half.

Patient #5
Condition: Diabetes Type II
Onset of Diabetes: 2 years
Pharmacological Treatment: For NIDDM, Glyburide 5 mg b.i.d.
Natural Medicine: Jambul combo 3 pills t.i.d.
Fasting blood sugar/Other indications: Before the study fasting blood sugar levels were around 12 mmol/L (216 mg/dL) and after the study were 10 to 12 mmol/L (180-216 mg/dL). The patient also had an increase in Glyburide from two pills two times per day to two pills three times a day,

again with no effect. The patient did not respond to natural therapeutics or pharmacological agents. It is interesting to note that this patient's was thin, while all the other patients in this study were obese.

Patient #6
Condition: Hyperinsulinemia
Onset of Hyperinsulinemia: 2 years
Pharmacological Treatment: Metformin 2 pills b.i.d.
Natural Medicine: Jambul combo 3 pills t.i.d.
Fasting Insulin Levels/Other Indications: Before the study, the patient's fasting insulin level was 36.8 u/ml. After 3 months of taking the herbal formula, her levels dropped to 28.7 u/ml. Within 2 weeks, she had noticed symptomatic relief. A rash that she attributed to the hyperinsulinemia had subsided. She stated that she felt better within a few weeks of taking the herbal formula.

Patient #7
Condition: Diabetes Type I
Onset of Diabetes: 2 years
Pharmacological Treatment: Insulin.
Natural Medicine: Jambul combo 3 pills t.i.d.
Fasting Blood Sugar/Other Indications: Fasting blood sugar levels were completely normal before the study. After the study, no decrease of daily exogenous insulin requirements were noticed. Before the study, the patient required higher insulin doses after rigorous exercise. Afterwards, an increase in insulin injections was not needed after rigorous exercises.

Patient #8
Condition: Subclinical Hypoglycemia
Onset of Subclinical Hypoglycemia: 15 to 20 years
Pharmacological Treatment: None.
Natural Medicine: Jambul combo three pills t.i.d.
Fasting Blood Sugar/Other Indications: Before the study, fasting blood sugar levels averaged 2.2 mmol/l (40 mg/dl). After the study, fasting blood sugar levels rose to 4.4 mmol/l (80 mg/dl). There was a significant decrease in hypoglycemic hunger and the patient's frequent need to eat.

The patient also noted a significant decrease in sugar cravings. The patient had taken 500 mcg of chromium daily for the previous 6 months. She had not noticed any significant changes with the past use of chromium.

Patient #9
Condition: Diabetes Type II
Onset of Diabetes: 15 to 20 years
Pharmacological Treatment: Insulin
Natural Medicine: Jambul combo one pill t.i.d. During the last week of the study, the dosage was increased to two pills t.i.d.
Fasting Blood Sugar and Other Indications: Before insulin therapy the patient's fasting blood sugar level was 200 to 240 mg/dL (11.1-13.3 mmol/L). Fasting glucose level on insulin therapy was between 150 and 160 mg/dL (8.3 -8.8 mmol/L). Fasting glucose after 3 months on the herbal formula was (7.4 mmol/L) 133 mg/dL.

Patient #10
Condition: Subclinical Hypoglycemia
Onset of Subclinical Hypoglycemia: 10 years
Pharmacological Agents: None
Natural Medicine: Jambul combo 3 pills t.i.d.
Fasting Blood Sugar and Other Indications: After 3 weeks of taking Jambul combo, the patient did not need to eat as often, did not feel jittery when missing a meal, and noticed an overall improvement in how she felt. She had taken chromium before but never noticed any significant changes. The patient lost 2 pounds a week while taking the herbal formula.

Patient #11
Condition: Reactive Hypoglycemia
Onset of Reactive Hypoglycemia: 8 years
Pharmacological Treatment: None
Natural Medicine: Jambul Combo three pills t.i.d., 500 mg of vitamin C daily, and vitamin B12 injections monthly.
Fasting Blood Sugar and Other Indications: Before the study, the patient had to eat 6 meals a day to avoid hypoglycemic symptoms. Hypoglycemic index before study was 26; after the study, it was 8. The patient reported

significant improvements over the course of the study in feelings of shakiness, irritability upon missing meals, heart palpitations after eating sweets, dependence on coffee in the mornings, mood disturbances, fatigue after eating, general feelings of faintness, poor concentration, and forgetfulness. The only symptom that did not improve was food cravings. Before the study period, the patient noticed waking headaches relieved by food. After the study, she experiences only two waking headaches per week.

Patient #12
Condition: Diabetes Type I/II
Onset of Diabetes: 4 years
Pharmacological Treatment: GE NPH insulin 20 units at bedtime, fast-acting Humalog insulin at breakfast, 15 units lunch, 15 units supper. Progression of diabetes before study: started with hypoglycemics (sulfonylurea) for 1 year then switched to insulin.
Natural Medicine: Jambul combo three pills t.i.d.
Fasting Blood Sugar and Other Indications: Patient's blood sugars before the study ranged from 4-15. After the study, they were stabilized at a range from 4-10. Before the study, the patient's high reading would last for a day or more; after the study, he would only get one high reading in a day. He also experiences less tiredness since taking Jambul. His insulin levels have decreased 5 units each at noon and bedtime. Before taking Jambul, the patient's insulin levels were increasing with time.

Patient # 13
Condition: Subclinical Hypoglycemia
Onset of Subclinical Hypoglycemia: 6 years
Pharmacological treatment: None
Natural medicine: Jambul combo three pills t.i.d.
Fasting Blood Sugar and Other Indications: Initially, the patient reported increased hunger, which disturbed her as she was trying to lose weight. She was instructed to reduce the dose to two pills, three times a day. Following this, she found a marked improvement in her energy levels, so much so that she quit smoking during the study period. Initially, her hypoglycemic score was 28; after the study, it was 13. She experienced significant

decreases in irritability, headaches, and shaky feelings. The only symptoms not improved were related to memory, concentration, forgetfulness, and sugar cravings. No other side effects were reported.

Patient #14
Condition: Subclinical Hypoglycemia

Onset of Subclinical Hypoglycemia: 10 years

Pharmacological Treatment: None

Natural Medicine: Jambul combo three pills t.i.d. She also took a multi B-vitamin, magnesium, vitamin E, and deglycyrrhizinated licorice to treat her other conditions.

Fasting Blood Sugar and Other Indications: Patient's hypoglycemic score before the study was 28; after 6 weeks, it dropped to 13. She noted a decrease in dizziness, impaired vision when standing, sugar cravings, palpitations, and tiredness after eating. Her concentration problems were not affected by the treatment. She reported improvement in fibromyalgia pain, but this may be due to other factors. No side effects reported.

Conclusion
The Jambul combo was an effective treatment in 5 out of 6 patients with NIDDM after 3 months. Most NIDDM patients noticed effects within 2 months. The treatment was effective in all 5 obese NIDDM patients. The only NIDDM patient who did not respond to natural therapeutics was thin. He also did not respond to pharmacological treatments. One patient with hyperinsulinemia noticed a significant decrease in fasting insulin after 3 months of taking the herbal formula.

One patient with Type I/II noticed a decrease in fasting blood sugar levels after 2 months of taking the herbal treatment. One patient with Type I noticed no decrease in fasting blood sugar after taking Jambul combo for 3 months.

Six patients with hypoglycemia noticed a decrease in hypoglycemic score within 6 weeks. The Jambul combo was an effective treatment in 13 patients out of 15. It was not effective in one NIDDM and one Type I patient. Most patients reported decrease in diabetic complications and the progression of the illness itself.

Side Effects

One patient noticed an initial increase in hunger after taking Jambul, but it went away after a week upon lowering the dosage to two pills, three times a day. Lowering of dosage may be coincidental or not. One patient noticed gastric acidity upon taking the herbal formula more than 15 minutes apart from a meal.

Notes of Reference to Pharmacological Drugs

Oral hypoglycemic drugs, such as sulfonylureas, have no long-term effect in blood sugar control for about 20% to 30% of NIDDM patients. In a study of Glucophage treatment of 228 patients, glycosylated hemoglobin levels of patients started at 9.43, after 6 months went down to 8.30, and after 9 months went up to 8.72.

Other Recommended Medicinal Herbs

Essential Oils for Diabetic Neuropathy

Background

Essential or volatile oils are aromatic oils extracted from plants. The pharmacopoeias of the late Middle Ages through the 19th century contained several essential oils, and they are still used in medicine today. Eucalyptus oils, camphors, and menthols are active ingredients in over-the-counter medicines; several volatile oils are used in dentistry as solvents and analgesics. These extracts are common ingredients in perfumes, toiletries, and soaps. They are also used as flavors. The chemistry of these oils and their principal components is relatively well understood, and many of the components have been synthesized.

Traditional Applications

Essential oils are volatile hydrocarbons produced by plants, which account for most of their characteristic smell; their function in nature is largely unknown. Their use by humans traces vaguely into antiquity, where the oils were contained in various unguents. Steam distillation provided the first practical source of the oils and came into widespread use in the 16th century, at which time pharmacies distilled their own oils. The alchemists' retorts and reflux devices were often charged with herbs and spices, from which they gained returns of <0.5% of a volatile oil. The industry grew as the technology improved, with the main activity in the pharmacies and perfumeries.

In the 19th century, the chemistry of the various component oils was the subject of extensive study, and assays for these components were developed for quality control. The high point of use and appreciation of essential oils appears to be the first half of the 20th century. Guenther published a definitive series of monographs (*The Essential Oils*, Vol 1-6, 1948-1952) that is still in print. Recently, aromatherapy has gained fashion, and there is a revival of interest in the naturally derived oils of various plants.

Pharmacology

The most common chemical structure of the essential plant oils is an unsaturated hydrocarbon of general form $C_{10}H_{16}$, known as terpenes. Oxygen-containing compounds of the general formula $C_{10}H_{16}O$ or $C_{10}H_{18}O$ are the second most common class of constituents. The backbone of the terpenes can be divided into two isopentane chains C_5H_8, which are joined end-to-end in several configurations. Since the terpenes are six hydrogens short of saturation, they always contain a combination of double bonds and/or rings adding to three. Differentiation through isomerism, substitutions, ring-closures, and addition of functional groups gives rise to the thousands of individual components described to date. Moreover, many of these are convertible into each other, so some components are always present as mixtures. Enzymatic conversion has also been demonstrated, so the pharmacology *in vivo* is quite complicated.

Biological activity of the essential oils has been studied for numerous types. Early uses included anti-helminthic activity of American wormseed oil, antibacterial activity of wintergreen, antitussive and analgesic activity for eucalyptus oil and menthol, and the many uses of camphor. Numerous over-the-counter remedies for colds, sores, halitosis, coughs, and sore throats still use plant-derived essential oils as active ingredients. For example, Listerine contains eucalyptol 0.091% w/v, thymol 0.063% w/v, and menthol 0.042% w/v. The coumarins are a type of essential oil and their use as thrombolytic agents dates from the early 20th century. Bergaptine is a photoactive compound used in tanning lotions. Pyrethin, the active ingredient in insecticides from chrysanthemums, is derived from a bicyclic terpene Δ^3-carene by oxidation.

Geraniol, the chief constituent of rose and geranium oil, is easily converted into the monocyclic alcohol α-terpineol, the chief constituent of the oil of hyacinth, and into linalool, which as acetate constitutes the characteristic component of lavender oil. Longer chains of terpenes give rise to many common compounds, such as the squalene, the carotenoids, such as β-carotene $C_{40}H_{56}$, and cholesterol.

Geranium Oil

Clinical studies have shown that using the essential oils of geranium and clove topically can temporarily decrease neuropathy pain. One research trial compared three strengths of geranium oil (100%, 50%, and 10%) with a mineral oil placebo and Zostrix, a capsaicin ointment. Subjects with post-herpetic neuralgia and moderate or greater pain were recruited. The patients completed pain assessments at times 0, 2, 5, 10, 15, 20, 30, 45, and 60 minutes following medication.

Results
- Treatment with geranium oil produced a highly significant reduction in pain ($p £ 0.002$) compared to treatment with the placebo.
- The reduction in pain produced by geranium oil appears to increase as its concentration increases ($p £ 0.003$). The observed increase is roughly linear, but a formal dose-response function cannot be defined because of the subjective nature of pain intensity.
- These conclusions were true both for spontaneous pain and for evoked pain.
- The response of an individual patient to treatment with geranium oil was similar for spontaneous pain and evoked pain ($p £ .008$): those who experienced relief with one kind of pain also experienced relief with the other.

Conclusions
The trial demonstrates that patients with neuralgia experience less spontaneous pain when treated with 100% and 50% geranium oil than when

treated with a placebo, $p \leq 0.002$. The averaged pain relief across all evaluated patients increased with increasing dosage of geranium oil, $p \leq 0.003$. The same conclusions hold for the evoked pain (allodynia), $p \leq 0.0002$.

Approximately one third of the patients had major relief, with little or no pain remaining; another third had some relief, such as reduction from severe to moderate pain; and the remaining third did not experience any benefit from geranium oil. There were no significant adverse events from the use of geranium oil. Only four patients of 30 had any adverse reactions, all mild, which were either a transient rash that resolved within the hour, or a burning sensation in the eyes that resolved within minutes.

Generally, users of geranium oil have reported that relief is experienced within 5 minutes and lasts for between 45 minutes and 6 hours, depending on the type and severity of the neuropathy.

Other Clinical Applications

Healthcare professionals have reported that geranium oil is useful for the following conditions in addition to diabetic peripheral neuropathies:

- Shingles (Herpes zoster)
- Post-herpetic neuralgia (PHN)
- Reflex sympathetic dystrophies (RSD)
- Spinal compression pain, including sciatica
- Causalgias
- Radiculopathies
- Phantom limb pain
- Fibromyalgia
- Bell's palsy
- Trigeminal neuralgias
- Myofacial pain

Evening Primrose Oil (Gamma-linolenic acid)

Background

Evening primrose oil is obtained from the seeds of the evening primrose (*Oenothera biennis*). This oil is a rich source of omega-6 essential fatty acids, primarily gamma-linolenic acid (GLA) and linoleic acid, both essential components of myelin and the neuronal cell membranes. Commercial preparations of evening primrose oil are typically standardized to 2% to 16%

GLA (8% typical) and 65% to 80% linoleic acid (72% typical), with vitamin E. GLA is formed by an enzymatic reaction involving the delta-6-desaturase enzyme. The enzymatic activity of delta-6-desaturase has been shown to be compromised in patients with Type I and Type II diabetes mellitus. This may make GLA less available to protect the nerve cells and also reduce production of prostaglandin series PGE_1, which is anti-inflammatory.

Clinical Studies

Gamma-linolenic acid has shown promising results in the treatment of many types of diabetic complications in several human and animal studies. In one trial of diabetic neuropathy patients, which was double-blinded, 111 patients were given either 480 mg GLA or placebo daily. After 1 year, GLA-treated patients showed favorable improvement in subjective symptoms of peripheral neuropathy, such as pain and numbness, as well as objective signs of nerve injury. People with good blood sugar control improved the most.

In another double-blind, placebo-controlled trial of 22 Type I and Type II diabetic patients with neuropathy, patients received 360 mg per day of GLA or placebo for 6 months. Patients receiving GLA had significant improvements in all six nerve function measurements and overall symptom scores. GLA, however, had no apparent effect on glucose control parameters. Side effects from GLA consumption were mild and similar for patients receiving evening primrose oil or placebo.

Dosage

In trials reporting positive results, a treatment duration of 6 to 12 months was generally required. The recommended dose of evening primrose oil, based on these studies, is nine to twelve 500-mg capsules each day, based on 40 mg of GLA per capsule. Equivalent GLA doses can be calculated using 1000 mg of EPO capsules or other oil capsules high in GLA, such as borage or blackcurrant oil capsules.

Safety and Side Effects

The side effect profile for evening primrose oil was generally mild and similar to placebo in the clinical trials mentioned.

Green Tea
Background

Much evidence is emerging that green tea has many promising health benefits. Green tea catechins (strong antioxidants found in green tea) have been shown to promote weight loss, prevent a wide variety of cancers, lower cholesterol, and promote a healthy digestive tract. Because green tea offers a wealth of other health advantages, including decreased risk of cancer and heart disease, its consumption (or the supplementation with a green tea catechin extract) by diabetics or those seeking to prevent diabetes is indicated.

Clinical Studies
Thermogenic Effect

Green tea has a thermogenic effect, which means that it supports the body's ability to burn fat. A number of animal and human studies have confirmed the ability of green tea catechins to promote weight loss. In one Japanese study of healthy men, weight, BMI, waist circumference, body fat ratio, abdominal fat, total cholesterol, and fasting glucose were noted to have significantly decreased after 12 weeks of supplementation with 483 mg of green tea catechins per day. The body fat reducing effect of tea catechins was confirmed in a study of 82 healthy male adults. When green tea catechins were given as a tea-like beverage for 12 weeks at a dose of 690 mg per day, approximately 10% of abdominal fat was lost. Since this corresponds to approximately 6 to 8 cups of green tea per day, it is difficult for many people to ingest this level of green tea catechins without developing side effects of caffeine consumption. In this case, a standardized capsule of green tea catechins may be more convenient with fewer side effects.

The value of catechins supplementation was confirmed by a study that isolated their effect on health. The study measured the 24-hour energy expenditure and fat oxidation of subjects who each consumed green tea extract, caffeine, or a placebo in three separate treatments. The researchers found that the green tea extract enhanced thermogenesis and fat oxidation that wasn't explained solely by its caffeine content, concluding that the green tea catechins were responsible for the fat burning properties. They measured a remarkable 4% increase in energy expenditure of subjects over only a 24-hour period as a result of the green tea extract. This, in turn, has the potential to reduce body weight and influence body composition over the longer term.

Antioxidant Effect

Evidence to support the effect of green tea catechins as strong antioxidant compounds that may offer protection from diabetes or even play a role in its management is also seen in research on animals. One 12-week study undertaken at the National Taiwan University found that giving green tea to rats improved their insulin sensitivity and lowered their blood glucose concentrations. The rats also had an increased number of insulin receptors and a protein, GLUT-IV, which transports glucose molecules across cell membranes more efficiently.

NATUROPATHIC MEDICAL PROTOCOLS FOR DIABETES, PREDIABETIC CONDITIONS, AND DIABETIC COMPLICATIONS

⑩

For practitioners of naturopathic and allopathic medicine, we provide the following clinical protocols for treating patients with diabetes, prediabetic conditions, and diabetes complications. Patients can also bring these protocols to the attention of their healthcare provider in a spirit of cooperative education.

Type I Insulin Dependent Diabetes Mellitus

Approach

Lifestyle and dietary modifications enable Type I diabetics to more tightly control blood glucose levels. By combining these efforts with botanical medicine, dependence on exogenous insulin can be decreased. Naturopathic approaches to diabetic management also play an important role in reducing the risk of diabetic complications. Quality of life is vastly improved through the prevention of complications that can range from mild to debilitating.

While it is widely believed that all Type I patients will eventually require insulin for glucose control and survival, rare anecdotal reports indicate otherwise with the use of IV hydrogen peroxide, niacinamide, and neuropeptide injections upon diagnosis. There are a few reported cases of completely eliminating exogenous insulin with the use of naturopathic medicine. Patients can also often decrease insulin requirements with the use of herbal medicine.

Lifestyle Counseling

Stress Reduction: Chronic stress plays a major role in the development of IDDM and diabetic complications by causing higher cortisol and blood sugar levels. Lifestyle counseling, meditative practices, such as yoga, and especially thermal biofeedback-assisted relaxation training (BART) have been shown to reduce stress, thereby stabilizing metabolic functions, reestablishing efficient use of insulin, decreasing the requirements for exogenous sources, and making blood sugar control easier to achieve.

Dietary Therapy

Dairy Products: Cow's milk should be avoided because antibodies to cow's milk are speculated as a possible etiology for IDDM in some individuals.

Low-Glycemic Diet: This diet helps reduce spikes in blood sugar and results in more regulated blood sugar levels. Over-consumption of highly refined carbohydrates is associated with the development of diabetes and its precursor blood sugar disorders. Based on a measure of how quickly a food affects blood sugar levels, the glycemic index provides numerical values for foods and enables patients to make better choices for managing their blood sugar. See the Glycemic Index of Common Foods chart in Chapter 7, "Dietary Therapy."

Clinical Nutrition

Niacinamide: High does of niacinamide (25 mg per kg) have been shown to suppress autoimmune disease in recently diagnosed Type I diabetes. Cases of complete remission with this protocol have occurred. This protocol may cause remission of Type I if done within 6 months of the diagnosis. If no effect has been shown within 8 weeks, chance of cure is low. Patients should consider neuropeptide injections, a low glycemic diet, and herbs after the 6-month mark or after trying this protocol without success.

Hydrogen Peroxide: H_2O_2 (30% solution), IV 2 cc in 250 D5W, three times a week, will kill microbial causes of Type I diabetes. This dosage needs to be administered immediately after onset. Cases of complete remission with this protocol have been reported.

Dioxychlor and Sulfoxamine: Administered IV three times a week, Dioxychlor and Sulfoxamine will address viral causes of Type I diabetes. Clinically proven in large clinical trials for reducing viral load after 12 treatments. Available from Bradford Research Institute.

Neuropeptide Injections: Administered every 3 weeks, neuropeptide injections have been used in treating autoimmune disease very successfully. Animal studies indicate complete remission of Type I diabetes. Human studies show success in reversing other autoimmune diseases, such as rheumatoid arthritis.

Vitamin D: Low vitamin D status has been shown to be associated with a number of autoimmune conditions, such as multiple sclerosis. Since Type I diabetes is also considered to be an autoimmune condition, researchers have investigated vitamin D supplementation and found it was associated with reduced risk of Type 1 diabetes.

Botanical Medicine

Gymnema sylvestra: 2 grams daily helps stimulate insulin production. No cases of complete remission with this approach have been reported; however, it significantly balances blood sugar levels.

Pterocarpus marsupium: 2 grams daily helps stimulate insulin production. Clinical research indicates significantly reduced need for exogenous insulin. No cases of complete remission with this approach have been reported; however, it significantly balances blood sugar levels.

Camal tamala: 2 grams daily helps stimulate insulin production. No cases of complete remission with this approach have been reported; however, it significantly balances blood sugar levels.

Hemopathic Medicine

Autohemotherapy: Molecular mimicry happens in a variety of autoimmune disorders that are triggered by infections and other antigens, such as chronic prostatitis, adrenal disorders, and thyroiditis. Autohemotherapy is a treatment used commonly in Europe by clinicians as a tool in treating autoimmune disorders. This process involves taking the patient's serum and homeopathically potentiating it. When the modified blood is reinjected in the patient, it is speculated that the patient synthesizes antibodies against the original antibodies.

Conventional Allopathic Treatment

Type I Intensive Therapy: For intensive care in Type I patients, it is recommended to test the blood 4 to 8 times/day to assess blood sugar control before and after eating. The patient is asked to count the exact amount of carbohydrates ingested or use the diabetic exchange system to make exact estimates on insulin adjustments.

Intensive control (micromanagement) of blood sugar levels reduces the risk of developing or progression of microvascular complications. Although optimal control has been defined as HbA1c <= 6.5% by the American Association of Clinical Endocrinologists, striving for an HbA1c of less than 5% is better. HbA1c should be tested every 3 to 6 months.

To achieve good results, blood sugar needs to be measured consistently:
* Upon rising
* 5 hours after Humalog or R (if used before meals)
* 2 hours after meals or snacks if no insulin is taken before
* At bedtime
* Whenever high levels are suspected

Goals for Other Tests

Triglycerides	<100 mg/dl (1.13 mmol/L)
LDL cholesterol	<100 mg/dl (2.59 mmol/L)
Fasting glucose	<100 mg/dl (5.5 mmol/L)
Bedtime glucose	<100 mg/dl (6.0 mmol/L)
Urine Microalbumin	Negative
Urine protein	Negative
Liver function	Normal

Nocturnal Hyperglycemia Management: The risk of secondary complications is caused by high blood sugar at any time, regardless of day or night. One way to stabilize blood sugar during the night is to split the insulin dose into one dose before dinner and one before sleeping. The latter injection will cause insulin levels to peak at 5:00 or 6:00 in the morning. The levels will maintain through the night, and nocturnal hyperglycemia can thus be avoided.

Troubleshooting the Insulin Regime: Diabetics may often have difficulty in keeping the blood sugar in range. Certain foods, especially high glycemic foods (foods that easily increase blood sugar), exercise, and physiological or emotional stress can temporarily increase blood sugar.

If the patient is taking insulin and hyperglycemia is still occurring, it is important to look at these contributing factors:

1. Accuracy of the self-monitoring blood glucose test
2. Pharmakinetics of insulin (abdomen>arms>thighs)
3. Diet
4. Stress
5. Use of corticosteroids
6. Menses

Type II Non Insulin Dependent Diabetes Mellitus

Approach

Because diabetes Type II is usually due to insulin resistance, the peripheral metabolism of insulin needs to be the primary focus of treatment. Second, because there may be some inability of the pancreas to produce enough insulin, pancreatic tonics are of value. Third, because blood sugar is controlled to a certain extent by the liver and adrenal glands, treatment needs to take these organs and systems into account. Fourth, because obesity contributes to Type II diabetes, lifestyle and diet factors must be modified as well. Stress, which tends to contribute to or worsen most conditions, also plays a role here and must be addressed. In our experience, if patients take the necessary natural medicines, make lifestyle changes, and manage their stress effectively, most will be able to wean themselves off prescription drugs completely.

Lifestyle Counseling

Poor diet and lack of exercise contribute to obesity, which is associated with the development of diabetes and its complications. Healthy lifestyle modifications are necessary in promoting the long-term health of diabetics.

Dietary Therapy

Low Glycemic Diet: This diet helps reduce spikes in blood sugar and results in more regulated blood sugar levels. Over-consumption of highly refined carbohydrates is associated with the development of diabetes and its precursor blood sugar disorders. Based on a measure of how quickly a food affects blood sugar levels, the glycemic index provides numerical values for foods and enables patients to make better choices for managing their blood sugar. See the Glycemic Index of Common Foods chart in Chapter 7, "Dietary Therapy."

Hypocaloric Diet: Modern diets are typically over-abundant in calories. Restricting calories to a healthy level may decrease insulinemia and improve cholesterol profiles.

Green Tea: Studies have shown that the use of green tea extract decreases obesity by increasing fat oxidation. Although green tea contains caffeine, other properties, including catechin polyphenols, appear to be responsible for its thermogenic effects.

Type II Diabetes Nutraceuticals and Botanicals

These medicinal nutrients and herbs are recommended for treatment of Type II NIDDM. Chromium and vanadium are crucial.

Herb/Nutrient	Action	Dose
Chromium picolinate	Helps with insulin efficacy	600-5000 mcg daily, to the level that controls sugar cravings
Vanadium sulfate	Helps with insulin efficacy	600-6000 mcg daily
Oplopanax horridus (Devil's club)	Helps with insulin resistance; also an adrenal tonic	1 g daily
Gymnema sylvestre (Gymnema, Gur-Mar)	Helps stabilize blood sugar	1 g daily
Taraxacum officinalis (Dandelion root)	Contains insulin	1 g daily
Silybum marianum (Milk thistle)	Liver tonic increases Hepatic Insulin Sensitizing Substance; useful for insulin resistance	500 mg daily
Galega officinalis (Goats rue)	Contains biguanides found in Glucophage; helps with insulin resistance	2 g daily
Nopal opuntia (Prickly pear cactus)	One of the most effective herbs in lowering blood sugar and insulin resistance at high doses only	1 tablespoon of nectar (10 g) twice daily
Syzygium jambolana (Jambul seed)	Aids in decreasing hyperglycemia; also increases glutathione and superoxide dismutase antioxidant levels	1-2 g daily

Conventional Allopathic Treatment

Pharmacological drugs have been demonstrated to be effective in decreasing glycosylated-hemoglobin and in the complications of diabetes. However, great improvement still needs to be made in the ability of patients to achieve tight control of blood-sugar levels. Due to the amount of side effects, the use of oral pharmacological agents should be assessed when administering drugs to NIDDM patients. Both hyperglycemia and NIDDM pharmacological agents may cause tissue-damage; for example, kidney damage can be caused by hyperglycemia or by the use of Sulfonylureas and Biguanides. Thus, it is important to determine which is more damaging to the patient, hyperglycemia or drug therapy. There are many reported hypoglycemic deaths due to the use of oral hypoglycemics. Other adverse effects include jaundice, decreased RAI-uptake of the thyroid, weight-gain, chronic hyperinsulinemia, severe insulin resistance, and perhaps beta cell exhaustion. Thus, if mortality due to diabetes is to be decreased, advances in more effective treatments are necessary.

Insulin: Insulin is not usually recommended in obese Type II patients because it exacerbates insulin resistance. However, thin diabetic patients respond quite well and have decreased microvascular complications. One other concern is that the use of insulin can cause weight-gain, which is a problem in perpetuating insulin resistance itself.

Sulfonylureas: Sulfonylureas have the advantage over insulin. There are multiple formulations available that are effective and relatively inexpensive. However, following long-term use, they may affect extra-pancreatic functions, such as increased peripheral sensitivity to insulin and a decreased hepatic glucose production. Sulfonylureas are contraindicated in patients with liver, thyroid, and kidney disease.

Metformin: Metformin is the drug of choice for obese NIDDM patients. It also leads to weight-loss. Patients with diabetic neuropathy may have symptoms associated with both diabetes and a vitamin B-12 deficiency due to the use of Metformin.

Alpha-glucosidase Inhibitors: Alpha-glucosidase inhibitors have a significant effect on blood sugar levels, but patients may not be able to take them long term because of gastrointestinal side effects. They are relatively new and costly.

Hypoglycemia

Approach

An effective treatment plan for hypoglycemia must examine the control of blood sugar levels. By encompassing lifestyle and dietary therapy, as well as botanical medicine, a holistic perspective is of considerable value. Results are best achieved by strengthening the health of the organs involved in diabetes. Herbal protocols support blood sugar control holistically through support of the pancreas, liver, and adrenal glands – the combined organs of blood sugar regulation. These herbs can naturally increase endogenous antioxidants, such as glutathione and superoxide dismutase (SOD). Thus, they can be of great benefit in treating retinopathy, neuropathy, and nephropathy, the common secondary diabetic complications associated with free radical damage.

These herbs are not drugs that lower blood sugar; rather they are aimed at strengthening the related organs so that they function better and regulate blood sugar more effectively. The effects of herbs for Type II diabetes can usually be seen within 1 to 8 months. Although these herbs are most helpful for lowering high blood sugar levels, they are also helpful in patients with low blood sugar.

Lifestyle Counseling

Stress: Stress plays a role in improper carbohydrate metabolism. Stress causes cortisol levels to rise, which can lead to decreased utilization of blood glucose and increased obesity and reactive hypoglycemia. If stress is persistent, the adrenals can become fatigued, which is also a major contributor to hypoglycemia. Because the adrenal response is triggered by low blood glucose, hypoglycemia exacerbates adrenal fatigue, as do simple carbohydrates (especially sweets and alcohol) and stimulant consumption. Therefore, managing stress, avoiding all stimulants, and supporting the adrenals will improve hypoglycemia symptoms.

Liver Support and Detoxification: The liver also plays a role in glucose metabolism, responsible for converting stored glycogen to glucose if blood sugar drops too low. Therefore, liver support and detoxification may improve the tendency to hypoglycemia by strengthening the ability of the liver to respond to low blood sugar. Thus, reducing toxic load on the liver by eating pesticide free foods and by avoiding chemical exposures (including over medicating) can improve the stability of blood glucose levels.

Exercise: Exercise has a number of benefits in the management of hypoglycemia. Exercise balances blood glucose by optimizing glucose uptake at the cellular level. Therefore, hyperinsulinemia is less likely to develop in a fit person. In addition, regular exercise balances the stress hormones and supports the adrenals, both of which help to maintain balanced blood sugar.

Clinical Nutrition

Alpha-lipoic acid: This amino acid is manufactured by the body and can be found in the mitochondria. Lipoic acid is a potent antioxidant that neutralizes free radicals and enhances the effectiveness of vitamin C and E, as well as sustaining blood sugar levels. It improves blood flow to peripheral nerves and may stimulate the regeneration of nerve fibers, which is very helpful to patients with diabetic neuropathy.

Hypoglycemic Nutraceuticals

These medicinal nutrients are also recommended for treatment of hypoglycemia. Again, chromium and vanadium are crucial, as well as alpha-lipoic acid.

Name	Indications	Pharmacology	Dose
Chromium picolinate	Insulin resistance	Improves insulin efficiency, which lowers blood sugar levels. Facilitates glucose uptake into cells as part of "glucose tolerance factor"	50-5000 mcg daily

Name	Indications	Pharmacology	Dose
Vanadium sulfate	Insulin resistance	Improves insulin efficiency, which lowers blood sugar levels	200-800 mcg daily
Alpha-lipoic acid	Insulin resistance Diabetic neuropathy	Decreases secondary glycosylation Excellent antioxidant	300-1000 mg daily
Pantothenic acid	Adrenal fatigue	Helps with adrenal support	1 g daily
Vitamin B-12	Neuropathy	Decreases diabetic neuropathy	1000 mcg daily
Vitamin B-6	Neuropathy	Decreases diabetic neuropathy	50-100 mg daily
Taurine	Hypoinsulinemia	Aids in the release of insulin	1-3 g daily
L-carnitine	Insulin resistance	Aids in mobilizing fat	1-3 g daily
Grape seed extract	Complications due to poor microvascular circulation	Decreases secondary complications; excellent antioxidant	200-800 grams daily
Quercitin	Cataracts	Aldose reductase inhibitor, antioxidant; decreases the accumulation of toxic polyols	300-1000 mg daily
Borage, evening primrose, flaxseed, fish oils	Dyslipidemia Neuropathy (EPO)	Help decrease blood sugar	1 table-spoon a day
Niacinamide	Protects islet cells of the pancreas	Helps with DM Type I autoimmune process if taken within first 6 months of diagnosis	25 mg per kg

Botanical Medicine

Gymnema sylvestre: This herb, used in India for over 2000 years to treat diabetes, contains a compound called gymnemic acid that has been shown to support the beta cells. It is a good herbal remedy for both diabetes and hypoglycemia. By supporting pancreatic function, *gymnema sylvestre* is helpful for both high and low blood sugar.

Eleutherococcus senticosus **(Siberian ginseng) and** *Panax* **ginseng:** These adaptogenic botanicals are also very useful for sustaining healthy blood sugar levels. Adaptogens increase the body's non-specific resistance to a whole range of physical, mental, and biological factors, allowing the body to deal with stress and adapt to change.

Glycyrrhiza glabra (licorice root): This herb inhibits the half-life of cortisol by inhibiting its peripheral breakdown. Hypoglyemia is often associated with adrenocorticoid insufficiency or low cortisol levels. Licorice is an excellent remedy for hypoglycemia because it helps to maintain cortisol levels.

Clinical Studies: Botanical Combination for Hypoglycemia

One clinical trial using 650 mg of herbal capsules three times a day consisting off jambul seed, prickly pear cactus, devil's club, milk thistle, and globe artichoke resulted in lowered fasting blood sugar levels by 33% in the majority of adult onset diabetics, while also raising blood sugar levels in patients with reactive hypoglycemia.

Hypoglycemic Score: Hypoglycemic patients were able to lower their hypoglycemic score index by 67% after 6 weeks administration of this formula. The hypoglycemic score is calculated by assigning a numerical value to the intensity and frequency of the following symptoms.

1.   Dizziness when standing up suddenly
2.   Loss of vision when standing suddenly
3.   Craving sweets
4.   Headaches relieved by eating sweets
5.   Feeling shaky or jittery
6.   Irritability if a meal is missed
7.   Heart palpitations after eating sweets

Hypoglycemia Botanicals

These medicinal herbs are highly recommended for prevention and treatment of hypoglycemia.

Herb/Nutrient	Action	Dose
Gymnema sylvestre (Gymnema, Gur-Mar)	Helps stabilize blood sugar	1 g daily
Eleutherococcus senticosus (Siberian Ginseng)	Used in China for fatigue, weakness, depression, forgetfulness, and insomnia; known in the West for its adrenal and liver tonic properties	2-4 g three times daily or 100-200 mg of a 1:20 extract (1% eleuthero-sides)
Glycyrrhiza glabra (Licorice root)	Prolongs the half-life of cortisol, thereby helping maintain consistency of blood glucose levels Antistress and antifatigue properties	1-2 g root three times or 250-500mg extract twice daily Should be used with caution in patients with high blood pressure
Oplopanax horridus (Devil's club)	Adrenal tonic that has demonstrated a specific positive effect in achieving blood sugar balance	1 g daily
Astragalus membranaceus (Chinese milk vetch)	Hypoglycemic	2-6 g daily
Silybum marianum (Milk thistle)	Liver support	70-210 mg silymarin three times daily

Adaptogenic Botanicals

These herbs have adaptogenic properties that increase the body's non-specific resistance to a whole range of physical, mental, and biological factors, allowing the body to deal with stress and adapt to change.

Name	Indications	Pharmacology	Dose
Allium cepa (Onion)	Hypoglycemic Antibacterial Antifungal	Competes with insulin for insulin degradation; increases half life of insulin	5-30 drops of fluid extract twice daily
Momordica charantia (Bitter melon)	Hypoglycemic Antibacterial Antifungal	Contains charantin (steroid) that decreases blood sugar; increases secretion and activity of insulin	5-30 drops of fluid extract twice daily
Trigonella foenum graecum (Fenugreek)	Hypoglycemic Digestive stimulant	Stimulates pancreas to produce more in insulin	5-30 drops of fluid extract twice daily
Syzygium jambolana (Jambul seed)	Hypoglycemic Digestive stimulant Excellent antioxidant Helps with diabetic secondary complications	Prevents conversion of starch and CHO into sugars; increases superoxide dismutase and glutathione levels	5-30 GTT of fluid extract twice daily
Pterocarpus marsupium (Kino)	Hypoglycemic	Prevents toxin induced B cell damage on the pancreas; helps regeneration in the pancreas; might be contraindicated in hyperinsulinemia patients	5-30 drops of fluid extract twice daily

8. Need to drink coffee to get started in the morning
9. Impatient, moody, nervous
10. Feeling faint
11. Forgetfulness
12. Calmer after eating
13. Poor concentration

Results: Since hypoglycemic patients often have a hard time coping with their hunger between meals when the blood sugar drops, they are likely to eat often. Most of the hypoglycemic patients who took herbs during the study had decreased appetite between meals; thus, patients were also able to lose weight. The study showed that herbs, when formulated holistically to address all the organs involved in blood sugar metabolism, not only are effective in addressing problems of high blood sugar but also problems of low blood sugar. Thus, it was shown that many of the herbs that were used traditionally to treat diabetes are also effective in treating low blood sugar levels, reinforcing the theory that some herbs have a regulating effect.

Conventional Allopathic Treatment

Conventional treatment for reactive hypoglycemia is limited because often it is not considered a real condition unless it is found to be secondary to pathologies known to affect blood sugar levels, such as:

1. Alimentary hypoglycemia caused by previous gastrointestinal surgery and peptic ulcer disease.
2. Hormonal causes, such early onset of diabetes Type II, hyperthyroidism, cortisol, epinephrine, thyroid hormone, glucagon, or growth hormone deficiency.
3. Endocrine conditions, such as insulinoma or deficiency of insulin receptor autoantibodies.

Conventional treatment for these conditions would be dealt with by treating the underlying cause.

Hyperinsulinemia

Approach

Hyperinsulinemia is often a precursor to Type II diabetes. In an effort to compensate for insulin resistance, the pancreas manufactures and secretes excessive amounts of insulin. Insulin levels become elevated *before* blood glucose levels are elevated, rather than in response to them. Prevention and treatment protocols focus on controlling insulin secretion. Hyperinsulinemia can be treated in the same way as Type II diabetes, with lifestyle counseling, exercise, dietary therapy, nutrient supplements, and botanical medicines. Hormone supplementation has been proven to help control hyperinsulinemia.

Clinical Nutrition

Hormone Supplements (Sustained Release T3 or WT3 Therapy): Many patients with Type II diabetes and hyperinsulinemia have low body temperatures and can benefit from sustained T3 release (Wilson's Temperature Syndrome T3 protocol or WT3). If the thyroid system appears to need help, WT3 therapy and/or other thyroid support can always be used. WT3 therapy has the advantage of not being needed to be taken for life, unless the patient has Hashimoto's disease. The improvements are often lasting, but WT3 alone will not always normalize insulin levels. Increasing body temperature is, however, indicative of increasing metabolism, which results in increased uptake of glucose of the cells.

Hyperinsulinemia Hormone Supplements		
Hormone/ Drug	*Indication*	*Pharmacology*
Pregnenolone	Adrenal tonic	Low adrenal function is associated with hypometabolism causing weight gain
DHEA	Adrenal tonic	Low levels associated with dysglycemia
Liothyronine	WT3 protocol helps with euthyroid and hypothyroidism	Low thyroid function causes weight gain and decreases insulin receptivity

Caution: Thyroid hormone supplementation can cause potentially lethal cardiac consequences in diabetics. Due to the increased cardiovascular risk, caution should be used when administering thyroid hormones.

Syndrome X

Approach

This metabolic syndrome of hyperinsulinemia is associated with high blood pressure, high triglyceride levels, and low HDL ('good' cholesterol) levels. Predisposing factors include a family history of Type II diabetes, a diet high in carbohydrates, and a sedentary lifestyle. Truncal obesity, fatty liver, difficulty losing weight, and hypoglycemia often accompany this condition.

Naturopathic Treatment

Syndrome X, like hyperinsulinemia, can be treated in the same way as Type II diabetes, with lifestyle counseling, dietary therapy, nutrient supplements, and botanical medicines. Exercise is proven to reduce insulin imbalances.

Conventional Treatment

Metformin (Glyburide) is commonly prescribed for insulin resistance in syndrome X and hyperinsulinemia. Metformin causes the liver to decrease its production of glucose, so that there is no longer excessive glucose to trigger unneeded insulin secretion.

Diabetic Retinopathy

Approach

Chronic diabetic retinopathy is very well treated with natural medicine by inhibiting the sorbitol pathway and saturating the eyes with antioxidants. Retinal hemorrhage is harder to treat naturally, but at times can be cured with the use of high doses of antioxidants.

Clinical Nutrition

Antioxidants: Naturopathic treatment of diabetic retinopathy involves the administration of high doses of antioxidants, including super oxide dismutase and glutathione IV, as well as herbs that decrease diabetic complications, such as jambul and milk thistle. Blue-light therapy has shown to be helpful in eliminating edema.

Botanical Medicine

Aldose reductase inhibitors: Aldose reductase inhibitors, such as quercetin and milk thistle, are valuable tools in preventing sorbitol production. Diabetic rats given aldose reductase inhibitors have shown higher concentrations of glutathione reductase than diabetic rats that do not have aldose reductase inhibitors. Botanicals, such as jambul and milk thistle, have been found to increase the production of antioxidants, such as glutathione reductase and superoxide dismutase.

Conventional Treatment

Conventional therapies for diabetic retinopathy are primarily control measures to stop the hemorrhage by using laser therapy.

Clinical Study: Diabetic Retinopathy

While conventional medicine is typically used to treat diabetic hemorrhage in the eye, naturopathic treatments have proven to be effective. A man in his mid-fifties with diabetic hemorrhage in the right eye visited our office for treatment. The right eye was 20/50.

We prescribed the following nutritional and botanical therapy:

- Ambrotose: 1/2 tsp t.i.d.
- Bioflavonoids: 500 mg t.i.d.
- Vitamin C: 500 mg t.i.d.
- Digestive enzymes: 1 per meal
- Dioscorea: 500 mg t.i.d.
- Vitamin E: 400 IU t.i.d.
- Bilberry: 500 mg t.i.d.
- Glutathione: 5 mg sublingually t.i.d.

Within 2 1/2 months, there was no more hemorrhage, and the right eye was 20/20.

Diabetic Neuropathy

Approach

The most common type of neuropathy is distal symmetrical polyneuropathy, which involves loss of vibration in the toes and loss of ankle reflexes. This can be found on a routine physical exam. Symptoms include numbness and paresthesias that may cause severe burning and prickling sensations. Pathological examination shows axonal destruction due to the complications of sorbitol buildup. Mononeuropathies come on with a sudden onset and leave usually spontaneously. They may affect the third, fourth, sixth, and seventh cranial nerve. Truncal neuropathy in the T4 -T12 area also exists. The pain is constant, unrelenting, worse at night, and is often confused with cardiac or gastrointestinal disease.

Many drugs inhibit the absorption of vitamin B-12 and can cause vitamin deficiency-induced neuropathy that must be differentiated from hyperglycemia-induced neuropathy. Neuropathy and vascular disease account for the high incidence of diabetic foot amputations. Diabetic neuropathic cachexia involves neuropathy along with symptoms of anorexia and depression. Autonomic neuropathy, including both sympathetic and parasympathetic nerves, can cause a variety of problems, including resting tachycardia, postural hypotension, bladder dysfunction, and lack of peristalsis in the stomach (gastroparesis).

Clinical Nutrition

Pyridoxine and Vitamin B-12: High doses of pyridoxine (100 mg) and vitamin B-12 (1000 mcg) can improve nerve function.

Vitamin E and Alpha-lipoic acid: Vitamin E at doses of 800 IU or higher, along with lipoic acid (300 mg), will inhibit protein glycosylation.

Quercitin: Quercitin at 2 g daily will inhibit the polyol pathway and give great benefit.

Botanical Medicine

St. John's wort: Clinically, we have found that one teaspoon of St. John's wort tincture, three times a day, relieves neuropathy and prevents progression of the neuropathy. St. John's wort is a nervine herb that can strengthen the health of the nerves. Patients usually respond within a week to this protocol.

Essential Oil of Geranium: This oil has also proven to be effective in decreasing neuropathy pain when applied topically.

Conventional Allopathic Treatment

Allopathic medicine has no effective treatment for diabetic neuropathy. Steroids and antidepressants have been tried with poor results.

Diabetic Nephropathy

Approach

End-stage renal disease, cardiovascular disease, and mortality are great risk for patients suffering from diabetic nephropathy. Nephropathy leads to systemic hypertension because of hyperlipidemia and a decreased clearance of atherogenic advanced glycosylation end products.

Diabetic Complications

There are five aspects that need to be considered in therapy for diabetic complications.

1. Hyperglycemia needs to be controlled as well as possible.
2. Free radical production in hyperglycemia needs to be quenched.
3. The polyol pathway in which excess sugar alcohols are produced needs to be inhibited.
4. The organs that are affected, such as the eyes, kidneys, and nerves, need to be supported.
5. Protein glycosylation needs to be inhibited.

Inihibiting Polyol Pathway and Free Radical Formation:

- **Quercitin:** 2 g daily
- **Vitamin C:** 2 g daily
- **IV Gluatahione:** 100 mg daily
- **Grape seed extract:** 100 mg daily

Inhibiting Protein Glycosylation and Decreasing Polyol Formation
- **Lipoic Acid:** 200-500 mg daily
- **Quercitin:** 1-2 g daily
- **Vitamin E:** 400-12000 IU daily

Infections

Approach

Diabetic foot infections are generally more severe and more difficult to treat than infections in non-diabetics because of impaired microvascular circulation, neuropathy, anatomical alterations, and impaired immune capacity in diabetic patients. Early detection and prompt attention by checking for signs of infection will significantly decrease the risk of serious complications. Neuropathy, not vascular insufficiency, is the main cause of diabetic foot ulcerations. Antibiotics and amputation are the conventional forms of treatment, but there are many naturopathic medical alternatives to pharmaceutical antibiotics. Simple natural treatments can go a long way in preventing and treating diabetic foot ulcers.

Clinical Nutrition

Inositol Hexaniacinate: This supplement is effective in peripheral vascular disease, including threatened foot amputations, gangrene, atherosclerosis, and hypertension.

Botanical Medicine

Horse Chestnut (*Aesculus hippocastanum*): This herb has a long folk history in venous support. It helps healthy circulation in the legs. It helps to control venous pressure, maintain vascular integrity, decrease damaging connective tissue within the vein, and prevent lipid peroxidation.

Green Tea: Adding 3 cups of green tea a day to the diet will significantly increase capillary strength.

Hydrotherapy

Hydrotherapy will also make sure tissues are being nourished by strong blood flow.

Ozone Treatment

Ozone treatment is an excellent way to treat serious conditions like this, especially when antibiotics fail. In one case, a 54-year-old diabetic with foot ulcer and osteomyelitis was told by his family doctor that his foot needed to be amputated. He opted instead for autohemotherapy and ozone therapy (limb bagging with ozone). After 10 treatments, he was cured.

Conventional Allopathic Treatment

Antibiotic Therapy: Antibiotic therapy often includes broad-spectrum antibiotics capable of covering the most common pathogens found in diabetic infections. Antibiotic therapy is nearly always active against *Staphylococci* and *Streptococci*, with broad-spectrum agents indicated if gram-negative or anaerobic organisms are likely. In infected foot tissues, the levels of most antibiotics are often sub-therapeutic. The duration of therapy ranges from a week (for mild soft tissue infections) to more than 6 weeks (for osteomyelitis).

Side Effects: However, antibiotic therapy, especially broad-spectrum antibiotics, can disrupt the normal flora of the gastrointestinal tract and vagina, leading to other symptoms, such as diarrhea, yeast infections, and thrush. In addition, other more serious opportunistic infections of the GI tract can occur, such as *C. difficile.* This infection causes frequent diarrhea, cramping, and mucous in the stool. It has been associated with deaths due to opportunistic infection in hospitals. Broad spectrum antibiotic use is also associated with allergic reactions in humans, an increase in antibiotic resistant bacteria, and disruption of the immune system. Some antibiotics have been shown to disrupt oxidative phosphorylation in the cell mitochondrion, leading to fatigue. Of course, there are situations when antibiotic treatment is necessary, but naturopathic treatments can still lessen or eliminate antibiotic use.

Antibiotic Alternatives

Like antibiotics, the natural treatments listed here should show symptomatic improvement within 2 days and need to be continued until 5 days after all symptoms have subsided.

Organism	Infection	Natural Treatment
Streptococcus	Cellulitis	IV Oxidative therapy
Staphylococci	Arthritis	IV Oxidative therapy
Candida	Thrush, urinary tract infection	Thyme essential oil, garlic
Klebsiella sp.	Urinary tract infection	Uva ursi, thyme essential oil, Mannose, buchu

Clinical Study: Diabetes and Infection

A 48-year-old woman visited our office complaining of fatigue and 'spaciness'. She had no history of any chronic health concerns. Upon physical exam, she was obese, had mild edema, and no flank pain. Considering her physical body type, insulin resistance and NIDDM is suspected. Considering her spaciness, it may be due to some blood sugar irregularity, her mild edema, and her debilitating fatigue. An infection is suspected. The lab results revealed a urinary tract infection, hyperinsulinemia, hyperglycemia, and hyperlipidemia.

The following three treatment programs were prescribed, with good results.

Program 1:
- *Uva ursi*, 1 teaspoon, with three drops of thyme essential oil every 2 hours for 3 days. This successfully treated the urinary tract infection.

Program 2:
- *Syzigium jambolana, Gymnema sylvestre*: 700 mg capsules, 3 capsules, 3 times a day.

- Dietary elimination of all simple carbohydrates.
- Blood sugar dropped 30% within 8 weeks.

Program 3:
- Inositol hexaniacinate, 1 g, three times a day for 3 months.
- Cholesterol and triglyceride levels were normalized after 3 months.

Clinical Study: Neuroinfected Diabetic Feet

A study at the National Institute of Angiology and Vascular Surgery in Havana examined the effect of various treatments on patients suffering from neuroinfected diabetic feet. Group one patients (15) we treated exclusively with ozone treatments, group 2 patients (13) were treated with simple cane sugar syrup (a traditional Cuban remedy for infections), and group three patients were treated exclusively with antibiotics. Treatments were analyzed to determine if they prevented amputation or if amputations was needed as the final resort.

Treatment	No Amputation	Amputation
Group 1 (ozone therapy)	93.8%	6.2%
Group 2 (cane sugar)	81.3%	18.7%
Group 3 (antibiotics)	66.7%	33.3%

Cardiovascular Disease

Approach

Diabetic patients have a fourfold chance of having both macrovascular and microvascular disease. Smoking, dyslipidemia, insulin resistance, homocysteine levels, emotional stress, and lack of general antioxidants due to the oxidation of LDL and low levels of vitamin E all need to be considered when treating diabetic patients with high cardiovascular risk factor.

The clinical signs of ischemic heart disease in diabetic patients are different than in other patients. Diabetic patients often will have a silent ischemia, making it more difficult to diagnose. Patients may have no pain, just nausea or sweating. Thyroid hormone therapy has to be used cautiously with diabetics due to its potential of increasing cardiac blood flow. Hypertension drugs can decrease insulin sensitivity, so whenever possible, natural medicine should be used in place of prescription antihypertensives.

Clinical Nutrition

Inositol Hexanaicinate: Inositol hexanaicinate works well in lowering lipid levels.

B Vitamins: Homocysteine levels also should be checked because high levels can injure the endothelial cells of the vascular system, resulting in increased platelet utilization and the formation of atherosclerotic disturbances, resulting in hypertension. One study found that men with very high levels of homocysteine were three times more likely to have a myocardial infarction, even while taking in consideration lipid levels. Homocysteine can be lowered with the simple addition of vitamins B-12 (1000 mcg), B-6 (50 mg), and folic acid (1 mg).

Vitamin E: Helps prevent protein glycosylation, thereby indirectly decreasing atherosclerotic hypertension.

Alpha-lipoic Acid: Also helps prevent protein glycosylation, thereby indirectly decreasing atherosclerotic hypertension.

Botanical Medicine

Snakeroot (*Rauwolfia serpentina*): *Rauwolfia serpentina* is a very reliable herbal treatment to lower severe hypertension. It is also an excellent remedy for anxiety and insomnia that often accompanies a hypertensive patient. However, like most prescription drugs for hypertension, some patients do complain of feeling tired when on Rauwolfia.

Hawthorne Berry (*Cratagus oxycanthus*): Moderate hypertension can be safely treated with hawthorne berry. It is extremely high in flavonoids that help limit atherosclerosis. It has the ability to help regulate tension, low or high, and is able to strengthen the heart muscle, as evidenced by clinical trials that analyzed the ejection fraction of patients taking hawthorne.

Traditional Chinese Medicine

Red Yeast: High cholesterol can be treated very well with the traditional Chinese medicine red yeast that contains at least nine statin compounds. Unlike its pharmaceutical counterpart, it contains only one statin isolate, and has no known history of causing liver disease.

Acupuncture: Acupuncture lowers blood pressure. Studies have shown that its hypotensive effects can last a year after the treatments have been discontinued. In contrast, high blood pressure drugs are difficult to stop once started because there may be a rebound in blood pressure.

Conventional Allopathic Treatment

ACE Inhibitors: ACE inhibitors are the drug of choice in diabetic hypertension patients. However, diabetics may develop severe complications with the use of antihypertensive drugs, including altered symptoms of hypoglycemia from beta-blockers, intensified fluid retention from sympathetic inhibitors, and worsened hyperglycemia from diuretics.

Lipid-lowering Therapy: Lipid-lowering therapy improves cardiac outcomes in diabetic patients. A study in Scandinavia on the use of statin drugs and diabetic cardiac outcome was assessed. The Scandinavian study was performed on over 4,000 patients. There was a 55% reduction in major cardiovascular events, including myocardial infarction, in patients treated with simvastatin. However, statin drugs have a history of causing liver disease, lowering CoQ10 levels, and leading to a painful and sometimes dangerous muscle condition (rhabdomyolysis).

Gestational Diabetes

Approach

Glucose control is critical. Optimally, pre-meal glucose should be less than 100 mg/dl with the 2-hour postprandial value not exceeding 130 mg/dl. Home glucose monitoring should be done at least four times a day. Mothers who achieve very tight control, as documented with normal glycosylated hemoglobin levels, have the same chance of fetal abnormalities as non-diabetic pregnant women.

Lifestyle Counseling

Exercise: Engaging in regular physical activity before and during pregnancy reduces a woman's risk of developing GDM.

Diet: Diet modification can also to help keep blood sugar level in the normal range while still eating a healthy diet. One way of keeping blood sugar levels in normal range is by limiting the amount of high glycemic carbohydrates in the diet. Eating smaller meals more frequently is helpful to balance blood sugars throughout the day. Skipping breakfast is definitely not a good idea.

Clinical Nutrition and Botanical Medicine

The use of minerals, such as chromium, and herbs, such as jambul, along with a diet avoiding refined carbohydrates, should be recommended. While oral hypoglycemic drugs are contraindicated in pregnancy, there have been no studies that have examined the effects of herbal hypoglycemics during pregnancy. Historically, most of the hypoglycemic herbs have not been contraindicated in pregnancy. They should be considered safe.

Secondary Diabetes

Approach

Secondary diabetes can be treated with nutrients and botanicals that support blood sugar metabolism and nerve, kidney, and cardiac function.

Secondary Diabetic Botanicals and Nutraceuticals		
Herb/Nutrient	*Action*	*Dose*
Inositol	Replenishes inositol depletion from hyperglycemia induced sorbitol osmosis causing inositol excretion	2 g daily
Vitamin B-6	Aids in neuropathy	100 mg daily
Vitamin B-12	Aids in neuropathy	1000 mcg daily
Coenzyme Q10	Aids in cardiac function	500 mg daily

Herb/Nutrient	Action	Dose
Alphatocopherol nicotinate	Improves blood rheology, decreases lipid peroxidation	300 mg twice daily
Aminoguanidine	Decreases advanced glycosylation end products	300 mg twice daily
Quercitin	Reduces aldose reductase	1 g daily
Anthocyanins	Increases capillary strength	180-215 mg daily
Silybum marianum (Milk thistle)	Antioxidant Reduces aldose reductase	1 g daily
Hypericum perforatum (St. John's wort)	Aids in neuropathy, both internally and externally	1 g daily
Eupatorium purpureum (Gravel root)	Aids in kidney function	1 g daily
Solidago canadensis (Canadian goldenrod)	Aids in kidney function	1 g daily
Vaccinum myrtillus (Bilberry)	Aids in eye function	1 g daily
Syzygium jambolana (Jambul seed)	Antioxidant	1 g daily
Cereus grandiflorus (Night Blooming Cactus)	Aids in cardiac function	10 drops twice daily
Convallaria officinalis (Lily of the Valley)	Aids in cardiac function	10 drops twice daily

Herb/Nutrient	Action	Dose
Crataegus oxycantha (Hawthorne)	Aids in cardiac function	60 drops twice daily
Leonurus cardiaca (Motherwort)	Aids in cardiac function	60 drops twice daily
Pelargonium spp. (Geranium oil)	Topical treatment for neuropathy (pain relief immediate but temporary)	topical
Ganoderma lucidum (Reishi)	Increases nitric oxide	1 g daily
Green Tea Catechins	Increases capillary strength	400 mg-1 g daily

Iatrogenic Diabetes

Approach

Virtually all non-controlled diabetic patients end up on antihypertensive drugs due to diabetic-induced high blood pressure, and many will need thiazide diuretics due to congestive heart failure initiated by the hypertension. Antihypertensive and thiazide diuretics drugs intensify insulin resistance, thereby further intensifying diabetic illness. However, antihypertensive pharmacological alternatives are available.

Botanical Medicine

Rauwolfia serpentina: *Rauwolfia serpentina* can lower blood pressure very well without affecting glucose intolerance. In Ayurvedic medicine, this herb has been used in the treatment of insomnia and schizophrenia since 1,000 BC. In China, it has also been used for thousands of years in the treatment of a Chinese pathology called 'liver fire rising'. Pharmacology studies indicates that it blocks the adrenergic transmitter vesicles, which take up and store the amines, resulting in depletion of norepinephrine, dopamine, and serotonin, and a consequent decrease in blood pressure.

References

A-D

Aharoni A, Tesler B, Paltieli Y, Tal J, Dori Z, Sharf M. Hair chromium content of women with gestational diabetes compared with nondiabetic pregnant women. American Journal of Clinical Nutrition 55:104-07.

Anderson HU, et al. Nicotinamide prevents interleukin-1 effects on accumulated insulin release and nitric oxide production in rat islets of Langerhans. Diabetes 1994;43:770-77.

Anderson RA, Cheng N, Bryden NA, et al. Elevated intakes of supplemental chromium improve glucose and insulin variables in individuals with type 2 diabetes. Diabetes 1997;46:1786-91.

Anderson RA (ed.). International Symposium on the Health Effects of Dietary Chromium. Published Online: 5 May 1999.

Anonymous. Intensive blood glucose control with sulfonylureas or insulin compared to conventional treatment and risk of complications in type II diabetes. UK Prospective Diabetes Study Group. Lancet 1998 Sept 12;352(9131):837-53.

Anonymous. Tight blood pressure control and risk of microvascular complications in Type 2 Diabetes: (UKPDS 38). UK Prospective Diabetes Group. BMJ 1998 Sept 12; 317(7160):703-13.

Babaei-Jadidi R, Karachalias N, Ahmed N, Battah S, Thornalley PJ. Prevention of incipient diabetic nephropathy by high-dose thiamine and benfotiamine. Diabetes 2003;52:2110-20.

Balch JF, Balch P. Prescription for Nutritional Healing. Garden City Park, NY: Avery Publishing Group, 1997.

Balon TW, Gu JL, Tokuyama Y, Jasman AP, Nadler JL. Magnesium supplementation reduces development of diabetes in a rat model of spontaneous NIDDM. Am J Physiol Endocrinol Metab 1995;269:E745-E752.

Baskaran, K. Antidiabetic effect of a leaf extract from Gymnema sylvestre. J. Ethnopharmacology. 1990;Oct 30:296.

Bergfeld R, Matsumara T, Du X, Brownlee M. Benfotiamin prevents the consequences of hyperglycemia induced mitochondrial overproduction of reactive oxygen specifies and experimental diabetic neuropathy (Abstract) Diabetologia 2001;44(Suppl1):A39.

Bishayee A, Chatterjee M. Hypolipidemic and antiatherosclerotic effects of oral Gymnema sylvestre R.Br. leaf extract in albino rats fed on a high fat diet. Phytother Res 1994;8:118–20.

Boden G, Chen X, Ruiz J, et al. Effects of vanadyl sulfate on carbohydrate and lipid metabolism in patients with non-insulin dependent diabetes mellitus. Metabolism 1996;45:1130-1135.

Borel JS, Majerus TC, Polansky MM, et al. Chromium intake and urinary chromium excretion of trauma patients. Biol Trace Elem Res 1984;6:317-26.

Borissova AM, Tankova T, Kirilov G, Dakovska L, Kovacheva R. The effect of vitamin D3 on insulin secretion and peripheral insulin sensitivity in type 2 diabetic patients. Int J Clin Pract 2003;57(4):258-61.

Borissova AM, Tankova T, Kirilov G, Dakovska L, Kovacheva R. The effect of vitamin D3 on insulin secretion and peripheral insulin sensitivity in type 2 diabetic patients. Int J Clin Pract. 2003;57(4):258-61.

Brown RO, Forloines-Lynn S, Cross RE, Heizer WD. Chromium deficiency after long-term total parenteral nutrition. Dig Dis Sci 1986;31:661-64.

Browner WS, Pressman AR, Lui LY, Cummings SR. The association between serum fructosamine and mortality in elderly women. Am Jour Epidemiol 1999;149(5):471-75.

Brunzell JD. Use of fructose, xylitol, or sorbitol as a sweetener in diabetes mellitus. Diabetes Care 1(4):223-30.

Buffington CK, Givens JR, Kitabchi AE. Enhanced adrenocortical activity as a contributing factor to diabetes in hyperandrogenic women. Metabolism 1994;43(5):584-90.

Buffington CK, Givens JR, Kitabchi AE. Enhanced adrenocortical activity as a contributing factor to diabetes in hyperandrogenic women. Metabolism 1994;43(5):584-90.

Buffington CK, Pourmotabbed G, Kitabchi AE. Case report: Amelioration of insulin resistance in diabetes with dehydroepiandrosterone. Am J Med Sci 1993;306(5):320-24.

Cardenas Medellin ML, Serna Saldivar SO, Velazco de la Garza J. Use of nopal dietary fiber in a powder dessert formulation. Arch Latinoam Nutr. 2002 Dec;52(4):387-92.

Center for disease control and prevention. Adult participation in recommended levels of physical activity – 2001 and 2003. Morb Mortal Weekly Report 2005;54(47):1208-12.

Chen TH, Chen SC, Chan P, Chu YL, Yang HY, Cheng JT. Mechanism of the hypoglycemic effect of stevioside, a glycoside of Stevia rebaudiana. Planta Med 2005;71(2):108-13.

Chiu KC, Chu A, Vay LWG, Saad MF. Hypovitaminosis D is associated with insulin resistance and beta cell dysfunction. Am J Clin Nutr 2004;79:820-25.

Chiu KC, Chu A, Vay LWG, Saad MF. Hypovitaminosis D is associated with insulin resistance and beta cell dysfunction. Am J Clin Nutr. 2004;79:820-5.

Chopra RJ, Bose N, Chatterjee P. Gymnema sylvestre in diabetes mellitus. Indian Journal of Medical Research 1928:16:115-20.

Clark CM Jr. The burden of chronic hyper-glycemia. Diabetes Care 1998;3:C32-34.

Crinnion WJ. Environmental medicine, part 4: Pesticides – biologically persistent and ubiquitous toxins. Altern Med Rev. 2000 Oct;5(5):432-47.

Crino A, Schiaffini R, Manfrini S, Mesturino C, Visalli N, Beretta Anguissola G, Suraci C, Pitocco D, Spera S, Corbi S, Matteoli MC, Patera IP, Manca Bitti ML, Bizzarri C, Pozzilli P; IMDIAB group. A randomized trial of nicotinamide and vitamin E in children with recent onset type 1 diabetes (IMDIAB IX). Eur J Endocrinol. 2004 May;150(5):719-24.

Cusi K, Cukier S, DeFronzo RA, Torres M, Puchulu FM, Pereira Redondo JC. Vanadyl sulfate improves hepatic and muscle insulin sensitivity in type 2 diabetes. The Journal of Clinical Endocrinology & Metabolism 86 (3):1410-17.

Dai S, Thompson K, Vera E, McNeill J. Toxicity studies on one-year treatment of non-diabetic and streptozotocin-diabetic rats with vanadyl sulfate. Pharmacol Toxicol 1994;74:101–09.

Davis W, Lamson, MS, Plaza SM. The safety and efficacy of high-dose chromium. Alternative Medicine Review. 2002 June;7(3):218-35.

Donath M, Gabor S, Yan X, Piva B, Brunner H, Glatz Y, Zapf J, Follath F, Froesch ER, Kiowski W. Acute cardiovascular effects of insulin-like growth factor I in patients with chronic heart failure. J Clin Endocrinol Metab 1998;83(9):3177-83.

Dulloo AG, Duret C, Rohrer D, Girardier L, Mensi N, Fathi M, Chantre P, Vandermander J. Efficacy of a green tea extract rich in catechin polyphenols and caffeine in increasing 24-h energy expenditure and fat oxidation in humans. Am J Clin Nutr 1999;70(6):1040-45.

E-I

Elkins R. Nature's Sweetener. Pleasant Grove, UT: Woodland Publishing, 1997.

Fagot-Campagna A, Pettitt DJ, Engelgau MM, et al. Type 2 diabetes among North American children and adolescents: An epidemiologic review and a public health perspective. J Pediatr 2000;136(5):664-72.

Fallon S, Enig MG. Nourishing Traditions. Washington, DC: New Trends Publishing, Inc., 2001.

Fawcett JP, Farquhar SJ, Walker RJ, et al. The effect of oral vanadyl sulfate on body composition and performance in weight-training athletes. Int J Sport Nutr 1996;6:382–90.

Ficarra P, Ficarra R, Tommasini A, et al. High performance liquid chromatography of flavonoids in Crataegus oxycantha. Il Farmaco Ed pr 1983;39:148-57.

Flora K, Hahn M, Rosen H, Benner K. Milk thistle (Silybum marianum) for the therapy of liver disease. Am J Gastroenterol 1998;93:139-43.

Freinkel N, Phelps RL, Metzger BE. The mother in pregnancies complicated by diabetes. In: Rifkin H, Porte D (eds.): Diabetes Mellitus: Theory and Practice. 4th ed. New York, NY: Elsevier, 1990:634-50.

Freund H, Atamian S, Fischer JE. Chromium deficiency during total parenteral nutrition. JAMA 1979;241:496-98.

Friedman M. Clinical study: Adaptogenic herbs in the treatment of blood sugar disorders. Toronto, ON: Naka Inc, 1998.

Frienkel N, Ogata E, Metzger B: The offspring of the mother with diabetes. In: Rifkin H, Porte D (eds): Diabetes Mellitus: Theory and Practice. 4th ed. New York, NY: Elsevier, 1990:651-60.

Gerstein HC. Cow's milk exposure and type 1 diabetes mellitus: A critical review of the clinical literature. Diabetes Care 1994;17:13-19.

Gharpurey KG. Gymnema sylvestre in the treatment of diabetes. Indian Medical Gazette 1926:61:155.

Goldberg B, ed. Alternative Medicine. Tiberon, CA: Future Medicine Publishing, Inc., 1997.

Gorio A, Donadoni ML, Finco C, et al. Endogenous mono-ADP-ribosylation in retina and peripheral nervous system. Effects of diabetes. Adv Exp Med Biol 1997;419:289-95.

Greenway F, Frome B, Engels T, McLellan A. Temporary relief of post herpetic neuralgia with topical geranium oil. American Journal of Medicine 2003 Nov; 115:586-87.

Greeske K, et al. Horse chestnut seed extract-an effective therapy principle in general practice: Drug therapy of chronic venous insufficiency. Fortschr Med 1996 May 30;114(15):196-200.

Gregersen S, Jeppesen PB, Holst JJ, Hermansen K. Antihyperglycemic effects of stevioside in type 2 diabetic subjects. Metabolism 2004;53(1):73-76.

Guens J. Stevioside. Food Chem Toxicol 1997;35(6):597-603.

Gupta SS. Experimental studies on pituitary diabetes Part II: Comparison of blood sugar level in normal and anterior pituitary extract-induced hyperglycemic rats. Indian J of Med Research 1962;50:708-14.

Gupta SS. Experimental studies on pituitary diabetes Part II: Comparison of blood sugar level in normal and anterior pituitary extract-induced hyperglycemic rats. Indian J of Medical Research 1962:51:716-725.

Haas EM. Staying Healthy with Nutrition. Berkeley, CA: Celestial Arts Publishing, 1992:98-101.

Halberstam M, Cohen N, Shlimovich P, et al.Oral vanadyl sulfate improves insulin sensitivity in NIDDM but not in obese nondiabetic subjects. Diabetes 1996;45:659-66.

Hammes H-P, Du X, Edlestein D, et al. Benfotiamine blocks three major pathways of hyperglycemic damage and prevents experimental diabetic retinopathy. Nat Med 2003; 9(3):294-99.

Hase T, Komine Y , Meguro S , Takeda Y , Takahashi H , Matsui Y et al. Anti-obesity effects of tea catechins in humans. J Oleo Sci 2001;50:599-605.

Haupt E, Ledermann H, Kopcke W. Benfotiamine in the treatment of diabetic polyneuropathy – a three-week randomized, controlled pilot study (BEDIP study). Int J Clin Pharmacol Ther. 2005 Feb;43(2):71-77.

Heikens E, Fliers E, Endert M, Ackermans G, van Montfrans. Liquorice-induced hypertension-a new understanding of an old disease: Case report and brief review. Neth J med 1995;4795:255-62.

Horrobin DF. The use of gamma-linolenic acid in diabetic neuropathy. Agents Actions Suppl 1992; 37:120-44.

Hypponen E, Laara E, Reunanen A, Jarvelin MR, Virtanen SM. Intake of vitamin D and risk of type 1 diabetes: A birth cohort study. Lancet 2001; 358(9292):1500-03.

Inzucchi SE, et al. Efficacy and metabolic effects of Metformin and trigladazone in type II diabetes mellitus. New England Journal of Medicine 1998 March 26;338(13):867-72.

Ishizuka T, Kajita K, Miura A, Ishizawa M, Kanoh Y, Itaya S, Kumura M, Muto N, Mune T, Morita H, Yasuda K. DHEA improves glucose uptake via activations of protein kinase C and phosphatidylinositol 3-kinase. Am J Physiol 1999;276(1 Part 1):E196-204.

J-N

Jack AM, Keegan A, Cotter MA, Cameron NE. Effects of diabetes and evening primrose oil treatment on responses of aorta, corpus cavernosum and mesenteric vasculature in rats. Life Sci 2002;71:1863-77.

Jacob S, et al. Enhancement of glucose disposal in patients with type 2 diabetes by alpha lipoic acid. Arzneimittelforschung, 1995 Aug;45(8):872-74.

Jacob S, Ruus P, Hermann R, et al. Oral administration of RAC-alpha-lipoic acid modulates insulin sensitivity in patients with type-2 diabetes mellitus: A placebo-controlled pilot trial. Free Radic Biol Med 1999;27:309-14.

Jamal GA, Carmichael H. The effect of gamma-linolenic acid on human diabetic peripheral neuropathy: A double-blind placebo-controlled trial. Diabetes Med. 1990;7:319-23.

Jovanovic L, Gutierrez M, Peterson CM. Chromium supplementation for women with gestational diabetes mellitus. The Journal of Trace Elements in Experimental Medicine 12(2):91-97.

Jeppesen PB, Gregersen S, Poulsen CR, Hermansen K. Stevioside acts directly on pancreatic beta cells to secrete insulin: Actions independent of cyclic adenosine monophosphate and adenosine triphosphate-sensitive K+-channel activity. Metabolism 2000;49(2):208-14.

Johnsen SP, Husted SE, Ravn HB, et al. Magnesium supplementation to patients with type II diabetes. Ugeskr Laeger 1999;161:945-948.

Jovanovic L, Gtierrez M, Peterson CM. Chromium supplementation for women with gestational diabetes mellitus. J Trace Elem Exp Med 1999;12:91-97.

Kalhoff RK. Impact of maternal fuels and nutritional state on fetal growth. Diabetes 1991;40;18-24.

Kano Y, Hirai H, Ito T, Kida K. Prevention of diabetes in non-obese diabetic (NOD) mice by short-term and high-dose IGF-I treatment. J Pediatr Endocrinol Metab 1998;11(2):267-72.

Kaufman FR. Type 2 diabetes mellitus in children and youth: A new epidemic. J Pediatr Endocrinol Metab 2002; 15 Suppl 2:737-44.

Keen H, Payan J, Allawi J, Walker J, Jamal GA, Weir AI, Henderson LM, Bissessar EA, Watkins PJ, Sampson M, et al. Treatment of diabetic neuropathy with gamma-linolenic acid. The gamma-Linolenic Acid Multicenter Trial Group Diabetes Care 1993;16(1):8-15.

Kilpatrick ES. Glycated haemoglobin in the year 2000. J Clin Pathol 2000;53:335-39.

Knight I. The development and applications of sucralose, a new high-intensity sweetener. Can J Physiol Pharmacol 1994;72(4):435-39.

Laakso, M. Hyperglycemia and cardiovascular disease in type II diabetes. Diabetes 1999 May;48(5):937-42.

Lafontan M. Fat cells: Afferent and efferent messages define new approaches to treat obesity. Annu Rev Pharmacol Toxicol. 2005 Feb 10;45:119-46.

Lahiri-Chatterjee M, Katiyar SK, Mohan RR, et al. A flavonoid antioxidant, Silymarin, affords exceptionally high protection against tumor promotion in the SENCAR mouse skin tumorigenesis model. Cancer Res 1999;59(3):622-32.

Levi-Ran A. Myogenic factors accelerate later disease: Insulin as a paradigm [review]. Mechanisms of Aging and Development 1998 May 1;2(1):95-113.

Loubatieres, A. The mechanism of action of the hypoglycemic sulphonamides: A concept based on investigations in animals and in man. Diabetes 1957;6:408-417.

Lupattelli G, Marchesi S, Lombardini R, Roscini AR, Trinca F, Gemelli F, Vaudo G, Mannarino E. Artichoke juice improves endothelial function in hyperlipemia. Life Sci. 2004 Dec 31;76(7):775-82.

Luper S. A review of plants used in the treatment of liver disease: Part 1. Alternative Medicine Review 1998;3:410-21.

Mahon BD, Gordon SA, Cruz J, Cosman F, Cantorna MT. Cytokine profile in patients with multiple sclerosis following vitamin D supplementation. J Neuroimmunol. 2003;134(1-2):128.

Majer M, et al. Insulin down regulates pyruvate dehydrogenase kinase (PDK) mRNA: Potential mechanism contributing to increased lipid oxidation in insulin-resistant subjects. Molecular Genetics and Metabolism 1998 Oct;63(2):181-86.

Mcdermott J. Endocrine Secrets. Philadelphia, PA: Hanley and Belfus Inc, 1998.

Melchior WR, Jaber LA. Metformin: An antihyperglycemic agent for treatment of type II diabetes. Ann Pharmacotherapy1996 Feb; 30(2):158-64.

Miyasaka A. Electrophysiological characterization of the inhibitory effect of a novel peptide gurmarin on the sweet taste response in rats. Brain Res 1995 Apr; 676(1):63-68.

Monnier VM, Kohn RR, Cerami A. Accelerated age-related browning of human collagen in diabetes mellitus. Proc Natl Acad Sci 1984; 81(2):583-87.

Murray MT. Encyclopedia of Nutritional Supplements. Rocklin, CA: Prima Publishing, 1996:88-99.

Naeser, MA. Outline Guide to Chinese Herbal Patent Medicines in Pill Form. Boston, MA: Boston Chinese Medicine, 1990.

Nagao, et al. Ingestion of a tea rich in catechins leads to a reduction in body fat. Am J Clin Nutr 2005; 81:122-29.

Nestler JE, Beer NA, Jakubowicz DJ, Beer RM. Effects of a reduction in circulating insulin by metformin on serum dehydroepiandrosterone sulfate in nondiabetic men. J Clin Endocrinol Metab 1994;78(3):549-54.

O-S

Okano H, Masuda H, Ohkubo C. Effects of 25 mT static magnetic field on blood pressure in reserpine-induced hypotensive Wistar-Kyoto rats. Bioelectromagnetics 2005 Jan;26(1):36-48.

Okuda K, Yashima K, Kitazaki T, Takara I. Intestinal absorption and concurrent chemical changes of methylcobalamin. J Lab Clin Med. 1973 Apr;81(4):557-67.

Olney JW, Farber NB, Spitznagel E, Robins LN. Increasing brain tumor rates: Is there a link to aspartame? J Neuropathol Exp Neurol 1996; 55(11):1115-23.

Orchard, TJ, Temprosa M, Goldberg R, Haffner S, Ratner R, Marcovina S, Fowler S. For the Diabetes Prevention Program Research Group. The effect of metformin and intensive lifestyle intervention on the metabolic syndrome: The

Diabetes Prevention Program Randomized Trial. Annals of Internal Medicine 2005;142(8):611-19.

Parillo M, Rivellese AA, Ciardullo AV, Capaldo B, Giacco A, Genovese S, Riccardi G. A high-monounsaturated-fat/low-carbohydrated diet improves peripheral insulin sensitivity in non-insulin-dependent diabetic patients. Metabolism 1992; 41(12):1373-78.

Pavlovskaya E, et al. Effectiveness of ozone therapy in the process of diabetes treatment. Abstracts: 2nd International Symposium on Ozone Applications. Havana: Ozone Research Center/ National Center for Scientific Research, 1997.

Petkov V: Plants with hypotensionsive, antiattheromatous and coronadilating action. Am J Chin Med 1979;7:197-236.

Pomero F, Molinar Min A, La Selva M, et al. Benfotiamine is similar to thiamine in correcting endothelial cell defects induced by high glucose. Acta Diabetol 2001;38(3):135-8.

Prince PS, Kamalakkannan N, Menon VP. Antidiabetic and antihyperlipidaemic effect of alcoholic Syzigium cumini seeds in alloxan induced diabetic albino rats. J Ethnopharmacol. 2004 Apr;91(2-3):209-13.

Prince PS, Menon VP, Pari L. Hypoglycaemic activity of Syzigium cumini seeds: Effect on lipid peroxidation in alloxan diabetic rats. J Ethnopharmacol. 1998 May;61(1):1-7.

Pyorala K, Pederson TR, Kjekshus J, et al. Cholesterol lowering with simvastatin improves prognosis of diabetic patients with coronary heart disease. A sub group analysis of the Scandanavian Simvstatin Survival Study (4S). Diabetes Care 1997;20:614-20.

Ravina A, Slezak L, Mirsky N, et al. Control of steroid-induced diabetes with supplemental chromium. J Trace Elem Exp Med 1999;12:375-78.

Ravina A, Slezak L, Rubal A, et al. Clinical use of the trace element chromium (III) in the treatment of diabetes mellitus. J Trace Elem Exp Med 1995;8:183-90.

Reljanovic M, Reichel G, Rett K, et al. Treatment of diabetic polyneuropathy with antioxidant thioctic acid (-lipoic acid): A two-year multi-center randomized double-blind placebo-controlled trial (ALADIN II). Alpha Lipoic Acid in Diabetic Neuropathy. Free Radic Res 1999;31:171–79.

Rosenbloom AL, Joe JR, Young RS, Winter WE. Emerging epidemic of type 2 diabetes in youth. Diabetes Care 22(2):345-54.

Rubin JS, Brasco J. Restoring Your Digestive Health. New York, NY: Kensington Publishing Corp., 2003.

Ruhnau KJ, Meissner HP, Finn JR, et al. Effects of 3-week oral treatment with the antioxidant thioctic acid (alpha-lipoic acid) in symptomatic diabetic polyneuropathy. Diabet Med 1999;16:1040–43.

Russell JW, Feldmen EL. Insulin-like growth factor-I prevents apoptosis in sympathetic neurons exposed to high glucose. Horm Metab Res 1999;31(2-3):90-96.

Sadri P, Lautt W. Blockade of hepatic nitric oxide synthase causes insulin resistance. American Journal of Physiology 1999 July;277(1pt1):G101-8998 and April;160(16):2377-81.

Saenz RT, Garcia GD, de la Puerta Vazquez R. Choleretic activity and biliary elimination of lipids and bile acids induced by an artichoke leaf extract in rats. Phytomedicine. 2002 Dec;9(8):687-93.

Schnaubelt Medical Aromatherapy. Healing with Essential Oils. Berkeley, CA: Frog Ltd, 1998.

Scorpiglrione N, Bellfiglio M, Carinch F, Cavalier D, Dekurtis A, Franciosi M, Mari E, Sacco M, Tagnoni G, Nicolucci A. The effectiveness and safety and epidemiology of the use of ascarbose in the treatment of patients with type II diabetes mellitus: A model of medicine based evidence. European Journal of Clinical Pharamcology 1999 June;55(4):239-49.

Shanmugasundaram ER, Rajeswari G, Baskaran K, et al. Use of Gymnema slvestre leaf in the control of blood glucose in insulin-dependent diabetes mellitus. J Ethnopharmacol 1990;30:281-94.

Shanmugasundaram KR, Panneerselvam C, Samudram P. Possible regeneration of the islets of Langerhans in streptozotocin-diabetic rats given Gymnema sylvestre leaf extracts. J Ethnopharmacology. 1990 Oct;30(3):268.

Shimizu K, Ozeki M, Tanaka K, Itoh K, Nakajyo S, Urakawa N, Atsuchi M. Suppression of glucose absorption by extracts from the leaves of Gymnema. J Vet Med Science, 1997 Sep;59(9):753.

Simoncikova P. Wein S, Gasperikova D, et al. Comparison of the extrapancreatic action of gamma-linolenic acid and n-3 PUFAs in the high fat diet-reduced insulin resistance. Endocr Regul 2002; 36:143-49.

Steinberger J, Daniels SR. Obesity, Insulin Resistance, Diabetes, and Cardiovascular Risk in Children. An American Heart Association Scientific Statement from the Atherosclerosis, Hypertension, and Obesity in the Young Committee (Council on Cardiovascular Disease in the Young) and the Diabetes Committee (Council on Nutrition, Physical Activity, and Metabolism). American Heart Association 2003;107:1448.

Stracke H, Hammes HP, Werkman D, et al. Efficacy of benfotiamine versus thiamine on function and glycation products of peripheral nerves in diabetic rats. Exp Clin Endocrinol Diabetes 2001;109(6):300-06.

Stracke H, Lindemann A, Federlin K. A benfotiamine-vitamin B combination in treatment of diabetic polyneuropathy.Exp Clin Endocrinol Diabetes. 1996;104(4):311-16.

Yu Sun Y, Lai M-S, Lu C-J. Effectiveness of vitamin B12 on diabetic neuropathy: Systematic review of clinical controlled trials. Acta Neurologica Taiwanica 2005:14(2).

Suresh Y, Das UN. Long-chain polyunsaturated fatty acids and chemically induced diabetes mellitus. Effect of omega-6 fatty acids. Nutrition 2003;19:93-114.

Swis Locke AL, Khuu Q, Viaole E, Wu E, Lopez J, Kwan G, Noth RH. Safety and efficacy of Metformin in a restrictive formulality. American Journal of Management Care 1999 Jan;5(1):62-68.

T-Z

Tager M, Dietzmann J, Thiel U, Hinrich Neumann K, Ansorge S. Restoration of the cellular thiol status of peritoneal macrophages from CAPD patients by the flavonoids silibinin and silymarin. Free Radic Res. 2001 Feb;34(2):137-51.

Toyoda K, Matsui H, Shoda T, Uneyama C, Takada K, Takahashi M. Assessment of the carcinogenicity of stevioside in F344 rats. Food Chem Toxicol 1997; 35(6):597-603.

Trocho C, Pardo R, Rafecas I, Virgili J, Remesar X, Fernandez-Lopez JA, Alemany M. Formaldehyde derived from dietary aspartame binds to tissue components in vivo. Life Sci 1998; 63(5):337-49.

Tuomilehto J, Lindstorm J, Eriksson JG, Valle TT, Hamalainen HH, Ilanne-Parikka P, et al. Prevention of type 2 diabetes mellitus by changes in lifestyle among subjects with impaired glucose tolerance. N Engl J Med 2001;344:1343-50.

Tyagi SC, Rodriguez W, Patel AM, Roberts AM, Falcone JC, Passmore JC, Fleming JT, Joshua IG. Hyperhomocysteinemic diabetic cardiomyopathy: Oxidative stress, remodeling, and endothelial-myocyte uncoupling. J Cardiovasc Pharmacol Ther. 2005 Mar;10(1):1-10.

Vaag A, et al: Is low birth rate, a risk factor for the development of NIDDM? Ugeskriept Laeger 1998 April;160(16):2377-81.

Van den Eeden SK, Koepsell TD, Longstreth WT Jr, van Belle G, Daling JR, McKnight B. Aspartame ingestion and headaches: A randomized crossover study. Neurology 1994; 44(10):1787-93.

Vasquez A, Manso G, Cannell J. CME Paper: Vitamin D (cholecalciferol): A paradigm shift with implications for all healthcare providers. www.alternative.therapies.com.

Vechi C, Tucci P, Galvin P. Chromium and diabetes: Relationship to serum levels of cholesterol, triglycerides and lipoproteins. Medical hypothesis 1980 Nov; 6(11):1177-89.

Velussi M, Cernigoi AM, De Monte A, et al. Long-term (12 months) treatment with an anti-oxidant drug (Silymarin) is effective on hyperinsulinemia, exogenous insulin need and malondialdehyde levels in cirrhotic diabetic patients. J Hepatol 1997; 26(4):871-79.

Verhage AH, Cheong WK, Jeejeebhoy KN. Neurologic symptoms due to possible chromium deficiency in long-term parenteral nutrition that closely mimic metronidazole-induced syndromes. JPEN J Parenter Enteral Nutr 1996;20:123-127.

Vieth R. Vitamin D supplementation, 25-hydroxyvitamin D concentrations, and safety. Am J Clin Nutr 1999; 69(5):842-56.

Von Schonfeld J, Weisbrod B, Muller MK. Silibin, a plant extract with antioxidant and membrane stabilizing properties, protects exocrine pancreas from cyclosporin A toxicity. Cell Mol Life Sci 1997;53(11-12):917-20.

Wagner H, Horhammer L, Munster R. The chemistry of Silymarin (silybun), the active principle of the fruits of Silybum marianum. In: Brown DJ (ed.). Herbal Prescriptions for Better Health. Rocklin, CA. Prima Health.1996;151-58.

Walton RG, Hudak R, Green-Waite RJ. Adverse reactions to aspartame: Double-blind challenge in patients from a vulnerable population. Biol Psychiatry 1993;34(1-2):13-17.

Welsh A, Eade M. Inoslitol hexanicotinate for improved nicotinic acid therapy. Int Record Med 1961;174:9-15.

Winer S, Astsaturov I, Roy K, et al. Cells of multiple sclerosis patients target a common environmental peptide that causes encephalitis in mice. The Journal of Immunology 2001;166:4751-56.

Winkler G, Pal B, Nagybeganyi E, Ory I, Porochnavec M, Kempler P. Effectiveness of different benfotiamine dosage regimens in the treatment of painful diabetic neuropathy.Arzneimittelforschung. 1999 Mar;49(3):220-24.

Wu LY, Juan CC, Ho LT, Hsu YP, Hwang LS. Effect of green tea supplementation on insulin sensitivity in Sprague-Dawley rats. J Agric Food Chem 2004; 52(3):643-48.

Xie H, Laut W. Insulin resistance of skeletal muscle produced by hepatic parasympathetic interruption. American Journal of Physiology 1996 May;270(5pt1):e858-63.

Xili L, Chengjiany B, Eryi X, Reiming S, Yuengming W, Haodong S, Zhiyian H. Chronic oral toxicity and carcinogenicity study of stevioside in rats. Food Chem Toxicol 1992; 30(11):957-65.

Yamauchi A, Takei I, Nakamoto S, Ohashi N, Kitamura Y, Tokui, et. al. Hyperglycemia decreases dehyroepiandrosterone in Japanese male with impaired glucose tolerance and low insulin response. Endocr J 1996;43(3):285-90.

Yaqub BA, Siddique A, Sulimani R. Effects of methylcobalamin on diabetic neuropathy. Clin Neurol Neurosurg. 1992;94(2):105-11.

Zhang JQ, Mao XM, Zhou YP. Effects of silibin on red blood cell sorbitol and nerve conduction velocity in diabetic patients. Chung Kuo Chung Hsi I Chieh Ho Tsa Chih 1993; 13(12):725-26, 708.

Ziegler D. Thioctic acid for patients with symptomatic diabetic polyneuropathy: A critical review. Treat Endocrinol. 2004;3(3):173-89.

Ziegler D, Hanefeld M, Ruhnau KJ, et al. Treatment of symptomatic diabetic peripheral neuropathy with the antioxidant lipoic acid. A three-week multicentre randomized controlled trial (ALADIN study). Diabetologia 1995;38:1425–33.

Ziegler D, Hanefeld M, Ruhnau KJ, et al. Treatment of symptomatic diabetic polyneuropathy with the antioxidant alpha-lipoic acid. A 7-month multicenter randomized controlled trial (ALADIN III Study). ALADIN III Study Group. Alpha-Lipoic Acid in Diabetic Neuropathy. Diabetes Care 1999;22: 1296–301.

Ziegler D, Reljanovic M, Mehnert H, Gries FA. Alpha-lipoic acid in the treatment of diabetic polyneuropathy in Germany: Current evidence from clinical trials. Exp Clin Endocrinol Diabetes 1999;107:421–30.